NATURAL EATING

Changing Your Relationship with Food

Charlton Hall, PhD

HOW TO USE THIS BOOK

Natural Eating is a 12-week program based on Intuitive Eating and on Mindfulness. Each chapter contains a weekly lesson plus a homework assignment. For the best results, read over the instructions and the lesson for each week, and complete the homework assignment for each lesson.

Contents

LESSON 1

WHAT IS NATURAL EATING?

If you're like me, you've had a life-long struggle with your weight. You've probably tried most of the popular diets. They worked for a while, then sooner or later the results tapered off and soon you were back to your old eating habits. It took me most of my adult life to figure out why. It's because dieting is about what you eat, but losing weight is about what you think about eating.

No matter what any of the diet gurus tell you, there's only one way to lose weight: Burn more calories than you consume. That's it. That's all. It doesn't matter what you eat as long as you don't eat more of it than you can burn off.

Of course that doesn't mean that you shouldn't eat plenty of fruits and vegetables and try to have a healthy diet. What it does mean is that an occasional piece of chocolate or ice cream isn't going to kill you. The key to eating whatever you want and still being able to maintain or lose weight is to remember the ONE RULE of weight loss: *Burn more than you consume.*

This means that as long as you keep the chocolate or the ice cream below your required daily calorie intake, you can still enjoy your favorite indulgences. One way to master this is to ask yourself, "Is one piece of chocolate more or less delicious than the entire box of chocolates?" In other words, it all tastes equally delicious. So do you really need to eat the whole box when one piece is going to satisfy you?

Key Concepts of Natural Eating

What makes it so difficult to lose weight and keep it off? The answer is that diets don't teach us to change our relationship to food. So unless we can also change the way we think about food, diets are destined to fail. That's why Natural Eating isn't a diet program. Instead, it's a program about changing your relationship with eating. Natural Eating is based on two key concepts: *Intuitive Eating* and *Mindfulness.*

Intuitive eating is a non-diet approach to your relationship with food. It works by helping you to become aware of how your body and mind respond to food.

Intuitive Eating was created by two registered dietitians, Evelyn Tribole and Elyse Resch, in 1995. It is a behavior-focused program that emphasizes what you think about food instead of on restrictive dieting rules. Intuitive eaters learn to listen to their bodies, which helps them to eat when they are hungry and to stop when they are full.

Mindfulness is simply paying attention to the present moment, with intention. Regarding eating, mindfulness is a way to get the most enjoyment out of every morsel, and a way to become more attuned to your body's signals so that you can distinguish hunger from appetite, practice intuitive eating, and learn to distinguish when you are full.

The 7Cs of Natural Eating

The key concepts of Intuitive Eating and Mindfulness combine to create the 7Cs of Natural Eating. These 7Cs are:

1 Cease the Diet Mentality.

Did your parents have a rule that you couldn't leave the table until you cleaned your plate? Did you eventually learn to feel guilty if you got up from the table without finishing every last bit of the meal? If so, you're like the majority of Americans.

We're taught to feel guilty about what we eat and when we eat it. Studies show that people who have difficulty with maintaining a healthy weight are usually emotional eaters. Guilt is an emotion, so when we feel guilty, we tend to eat more.

If we feel guilty for not sticking with the rules of a diet, we've set ourselves up for failure because that guilt is the very thing that triggers us to eat more.

Natural eating is about listening to what your body tells you. It's not about restrictive diets and their guilt-inducing rules. When we get to be in tune to our body's natural needs we're better able to change our relationship with food.

2 Conscious eating is mindful eating.

Have you ever sat down with a bag of chips and told yourself just to eat a few, then looked down to realize you'd eaten the whole bag? Are you consciously and intentionally aware of every morsel of food you put into your mouth? Are you always consciously aware of the difference between hunger and appetite? Are you always consciously aware of when your body is telling you that you're full? Conscious eating uses the skills of mindful awareness to make all eating aware eating. Conscious eating is about using mindful eating skills to feel more satisfied with less food.

3 Call a truce by allowing yourself to eat whatever you want.

The only rule about losing weight is "in vs. out." The key to losing is to eat less than you burn. If you can learn to eat smaller quantities of the foods you love, you can lower your calorie consumption rate, allowing yourself to lose weight naturally, without guilt.

4 Challenge the Food Police.

Diets tend to induce guilt. Guilt tends to lead emotional eaters to eat more. Natural eating challenges the food police by reminding participants that it's okay to eat what you want, and to listen to your own body's needs. Challenging the Food Police means not blaming, shaming, or guilt-tripping yourself when it comes to your relationship with food, and not allowing others to do so either.

5 Connect to your senses of hunger and satisfaction using mindful eating.

Mindful eating is conscious eating. When we teach ourselves to engage in mindful eating, we learn to distinguish between hunger and appetite, to recognize our bodies' signals that we are full, and to accept ourselves as we are.

6 Comfort your feelings, not your appetite.

Pretty much everyone on the planet has been an emotional eater at one time or another. We tend to seek comfort in food because it's one of the most basic necessities of life.

Natural eating teaches us to find comfort for our feelings in other ways than food. When we're able to do this, we naturally let go of the tendency to be emotional eaters.

7 Choose Change by increasing your motivation.

When does change happen? The only time change happens is when the pain of staying the same is greater than the pain of changing. The way to change our eating habits is to increase our motivation to change.

There are two ways to do this. The first is to increase the pleasure in changing. The second is to increase the pain in staying the same. If we do either of these things, we increase our motivation to eat in healthy ways.

Food Tracker

The first two Cs of Natural Eating involve ceasing the diet mentality and becoming conscious eaters. The place to begin with this is by being aware of what we eat on a daily basis. We're going to do this by tracking our food.

For the next 4 weeks, use a chart to track what you eat. For now, don't worry about making any modifications to your food intake. Just record everything you eat, no matter how small. Even if you only eat a single strawberry or one bite of chocolate cake, document it.

The reason for this is twofold:

1. To cease the diet mentality, you have to learn what you like and what you don't like;
2. To become a conscious eater, you have to be conscious of what your food intake is.

Use the table at the end of this section to track your food intake. If you are proficient in spreadsheet software, you may wish to create a spreadsheet to make tracking easier.

We're tracking seven things in this chart. What they are and why we're tracking them is listed below.

1. What you ate

This helps you to identify patterns in your food intake. Most people have at best a list of about 100 to 150 foods that they eat on a regular basis. The "Food Glossary" tab on the spreadsheet is for tracking the information for your list of favorite foods. When you can identify those patterns you can modify them as needed.

2. How much you ate

This helps you to identify the usual quantities (number of servings) of each food you eat at a sitting. This information can later be used to modify the foods you eat based on the 7Cs of Natural Eating if necessary.

3.   Total calories in what you ate

This helps you to identify your food intake in a given day. Remember that the only rule for losing weight is to eat less than you burn. Calories are what you're burning, so knowing your calorie intake is half the equation. The other half, knowing how much you burn, will be a topic for another day.

4.   Total protein in what you ate

Protein is the stuff that satisfies our sense of being full. The more protein per calorie of intake, the more full you feel. Tracking your protein intake helps you to establish your calorie-to-protein intake so that you can feel more full on less calories.

5.   Total fat in what you ate

Once you've burned all the calories and fat your body needs in a given day, the rest is stored in your fat cells. Fats don't require any additional processing by your body. If you've met your energy needs for the day, any surplus fat goes directly to your fat cells. Being aware of the amount of fat in your foods helps you to modify what you eat, should you decide to do so.

6.   Total carbohydrates in what you ate

Carbohydrates are "instant energy." They're turned into sugars, and sugars are used by your body to produce energy. Your body has to process them into sugars, so they do require a little extra work, but any carbohydrates your body doesn't burn are stored energy for later use. This energy is stored in your fat cells.

7. *Total sugars in what you ate*

Sugar is an addictive substance. Eating sugar stimulates your dopamine system, like most other addictive drugs. Tracking your sugar intake helps you to be conscious of the amount of sugar you may be eating so that you can modify the way you eat naturally.

FOOD TRACKER

DATE	FOOD	QUANTITY	CALORIES	PROTEIN	FAT	CARBS	SUGAR
SUN							
MON							
TUE							
WED							
THUR							
FRI							
SAT							

For the next four weeks, track your food intake on the table provided above, or create your own. Most pre-packaged foods have nutrition information on the package somewhere. For foods that aren't processed, or foods that don't come with labels, you may wish to use one of the websites in the *References* section below for nutrition information.

Food Glossary

If you're like most people, you have a selection of favorite foods that you most often eat. On average most people eat about two to three dozen different dishes on a regular basis. Because of this you may find it convenient, when tracking your food intake, to create a Food Glossary that tracks the nutritional information for your favorites.

You may then use this information as a matter of convenience so that you don't have to continually look up nutritional information for your daily food intake.

You can create such a glossary using a table similar to the one

Next week we'll talk about how to begin making the changes you want to make using intuitive eating and mindfulness.

KEY POINTS TO REMEMBER FOR LESSON 1

- The only rule to remember for losing weight is to burn more calories than you consume.

- The 7Cs of Natural Eating isn't a diet program. It's a program about changing your relationship with food.

- The 7Cs of Natural Eating is based on the principles of Intuitive Eating and Mindful Eating.

- The 7Cs of Natural Eating are:

  1. Cease the Diet Mentality
  2. Conscious Eating - using mindful eating to feel satisfied with less food
  3. Call a truce - allow yourself to eat whatever you want. The only rule for weight loss is to burn more than you consume.
  4. Challenge the Food Police
  5. Connect to your senses of hunger and satisfaction
  6. Comfort your feelings, not your appetite
  7. Choose Change - increase motivation using theory of change

REFERENCES

Avena, N. M., Rada, P., & Hoebel, B. G. (2008). Evidence for sugar addiction: behavioral and neurochemical effects of intermittent, excessive sugar intake. *Neuroscience and biobehavioral reviews*, 32(1), 20–39.

Nutritional Information

Use the websites below to track nutritional information for your *Food Tracker* and *Food Glossary*.

Academy of Nutrition and Dietetics

>   https://www.eatright.org
>   https://www.eatright.org/for-kids

>   *U.S. Department of Agriculture*
>   https://www.myplate.gov

If diabetes and diet are of concern to you, use the American Diabetes Association website.

>   *American Diabetes Association*
>   https://diabetes.org

If you have food allergies, there's a wealth of information on the FARE site.

Food Allergy Research and Education
https://www.foodallergy.org

Any of the sites listed above can provide you with nutrition information for most of the foods you eat. If you can't find what you're looking for on any of those sites, try an internet search instead.

LESSON 2

CHANGING YOUR RELATIONSHIP WITH FOOD

Theory of Change

There are a lot of theories about why change happens, but they all boil down to the following:

Change happens when the pain of staying the same becomes greater than the pain of changing.

Think about some times in your life when you made a change for the better, and you can probably readily identify the point when you made the decision that the pain of staying the same was greater than the pain of changing.

Change is hard. Sometimes when we make changes, the new way of doing things feels weird or strange. If it didn't, you'd already be doing things a different way.

Part of the difficulty of change comes down to having to re-learn how to do things. One way to learn a new way of doing things is to act out of conscious intention.

Intention is one of the skills of mindfulness that we'll cover in more detail in Lesson 4, but for now let's just say that intention means doing more of what works and less of what doesn't work. The way to apply intention to change is to act with conscious intention to either increase the pain of staying the same or decrease the pain of changing.

When it comes to eating, or changing the way you eat, you have two choices. You can focus on the things that increase the pain of eating the way you've always eating or you can focus on the thoughts and behaviors that increase the pleasure (thereby decreasing the pain) of making the conscious, intentional choice to change.

We'll be talking more about how to do this later on in this week's lesson, but for now let's talk about how change happens.

Stages of Change

According to the Trans-Theoretical Model of Change, change happens in six stages, if it happens at all. Let's review what these six stages are.

1.   Pre-Contemplative

This is sometimes referred to as the "denial" stage. People in this stage usually make statements like, "I don't have a problem." When a person is pre-contemplative, they're not likely to be ready for change. If you are participating in this Natural Eating course, it's probably safe to assume that you're already past this stage.

2.   Contemplative

In this stage, people are not quite sure that there's a problem, but they're at least willing to consider the possibility that a problem exists. They usually say things like, "I'm not sure if I have a problem or not, but I'm open to investigating."

3.   Preparation

This is the information-gathering stage. Once a person has decided that there is a problem, the next step is to determine what to do about it. This includes gathering as much information as possible about all the potential solutions to the problem. People at this stage say things like, "Okay, there's a problem. Now what am I going to do about it?"

4.   Action

Once all the information has been gathered, and all the potential solutions have been evaluated, it's time to pick one and implement it.

People at this stage make statements like, "I admit there's a problem, and here's my solution."

5. *Relapse*

This stage isn't inevitable, but it's included here because research has shown that people relapse an average of three times before making permanent change. For our purposes here, "relapse" means returning to old behaviors. If this happens to you, the way to deal with it is to troubleshoot what went wrong, modify your plan of change to incorporate the new information, and then implement the solution again with the new information.

6. *Maintenance*

Once you've engaged in troubleshooting, fixed all the potential bugs in your solution, and come up with a plan that works, you're in the maintenance phase. This means that you're able to continue implementing your change plan successfully by increasing the pain of staying the same while decreasing the pain of changing.

Statement of Purpose

So how do you go about increasing the pain of staying the same while increasing the pleasure of committing to change? The simplest way to do this is to first come up with something called a Statement of Purpose.

A Statement of Purpose for making Natural Eating changes is designed to increase the pain of staying the same (continuing your current eating patterns) and to increase the pleasure of making positive changes (changing your eating patterns naturally). This is done by completing the Statement of Purpose worksheet at the end of this section.

It is crucial that you complete your Statement of Purpose prior to the next Lesson in the program, as it is the core of the Natural Eating program. Without a Statement of Purpose it will be extremely difficult to make changes.

Here are some guidelines to use when filling out your Statement of Purpose:

Think about why you want to make the change. Is it for health reasons? For appearance reasons? For some other reason? List as many reasons for change as you can think of.

Next, for each item on your list identify where you are for that item on the Stages of Change outlined above. If you're contemplative or pre-contemplative for any item on your list, ask yourself what information would help you to get to the preparation stage. Then find that information and add it to your Statement of Purpose.

Finally, go through your list and note how many items on it are changes that you want to make for yourself, eliminating any changes you're trying to make because of other people.

Now look at the column labeled "Increasing the Pain of Staying the Same." Incorporating the information you gathered from the steps above, list as many things as you can think of that would help you to focus on increasing the pain of staying the same should you lose your motivation to make change. Some examples might include less energy, increased health risks, or not feeling good about yourself.

Then, in the column labeled, "Increasing the Pleasure of Changing," list as many things as you can think of that you could focus on to increase the pleasure of changing your eating habits should you lose your motivation to change. Some examples might be better health, more energy, or increased life satisfaction.

Once you have all this information written down, it may help to write it all out in paragraph form, or you may just keep the Statement of Purpose worksheet to refer to whenever you notice a lack of motivation.

NATURAL EATING STATEMENT OF PURPOSE

- Use the space below to describe why you want to change your relationship with food. Is it for health reasons? For appearance reasons? For some other reason? List as many reasons for change as you can think of.
- Next, for each item on your list, identify which stage of change you are in for that item on the Stages of Change outlined in Session 2 of the Natural Eating Program.
- Finally, go through your list and note how many items on it are changes that you want to make for yourself, eliminating any changes you're trying to make because of other people. If you are trying to make changes because it's what you think other people want you to do instead of what you want to do for yourself, it's going to be hard to stay motivated for change. The best way to make change is to want to do it yourself.

Why do you want to change your relationship with food?	Stage of Change for this item

MOTIVATIONS FOR CHANGE

In the column below labeled *Increasing the Pain of Staying the Same*, list as many things as you can think of that would help you to focus on increasing the pain of staying the same should you lose your motivation to make change. Some examples might include less energy, increased health risks, or not feeling good about yourself. Then, in the column labeled *Increasing the Pleasure of Changing*, list as many things as you can think of that you could focus on to increase the pleasure of changing your eating habits should you lose your motivation to change. Some examples might be better health, more energy, or increased life satisfaction. Once you have all this information written down, it may help to write it all out in paragraph form, or you may just keep this Statement of Purpose worksheet to refer to whenever you feel your motivation slipping. Use more paper if needed.

Increasing the Pain of Staying the Same	Increasing the Pleasure of Changing

Change Plan

Now that you have your *Statement of Purpose*, you're ready to move on to your Change Plan.

In Natural Eating, the Statement of Purpose is what changes you want to make, and the Change Plan is the roadmap for making that change happen. To simplify, the Statement of Purpose is the "what" and the Change Plan is the "how."

To complete your Change Plan, read over the information below, then use the Change Plan worksheet at the end of this section as a template to complete your Change Plan.

Follow the instructions below to complete your Change Plan. You may wish to create a hard copy and place it somewhere where you will see it every day, like on your bathroom mirror or on your refrigerator.

Instructions for Completing Your Change Plan

Some changes I want to make include…

In this section, use your Statement of Purpose to list some of the changes you want to make in your eating habits.

The reasons why I want to make these changes include…

In this section, list some of the reasons you listed on your Statement of Purpose. Alternately, you may just refer to your Statement of Purpose instead of completing this section. For ease of reference, you may wish to just pick the top two or three reasons from your Statement of Purpose that you wish to make changes and list them on your Change Plan in this section.

My plan for making these changes is to…

This section is a work in progress because as you progress through the Natural Eating program you will be learning new techniques and tips for making change, so you can always add to this section as you progress through the program. For now just list a few things that you already know would help you make changes.

I will know my plan is working when this happens…

Be as specific as possible when answering this section. For example, instead of saying, "When I lose weight," say something like, "When I lose 5 pounds." The more specific you can be in your answers, the more you increase your chances of success.

Some things that could interfere with my plan for change include…

Have you been on diets before? Have they been successful? If not, you already know from personal experience what some roadblocks to making change might be, so list them here as preparation for making a plan to prevent them should they occur again.

If those things interfere, I plan to…

It's okay if you don't know how to answer this section yet. If you do, great…list a few things here. If not, you can fill it in later as you progress through the program.

Use the scale below to answer the following questions

The three questions listed in this section help you to gauge your own motivation for change. As you rate yourself on each of the three questions, ask yourself what it would take to get the numbers a little higher for each question, then focus on doing just that as you progress through the program.

Change Plan Worksheet

Some changes I want to make include:

The reasons why I want to make these changes include:

My plan for making these changes is to:

I will know my plan is working when this happens:

Some things that could interfere with my plan for change include:

If those things interfere, I plan to:

Use the scale below to answer the following questions:

Not important at all – 0 – 1 – 2 – 3 – 4 – 5 – 6 – 7 – 8 – 9 – 10 – Very important

_____ How important is it to make this change?

_____ How motivated am I to make this change?

_____ How confident am I that I can make this change?

FOOD TRACKER

If you followed the instructions from last week's lesson, you should have begun to track your food intake.

In future lessons we'll be going into more depth regarding what all the information in your food tracker means. For now, the most significant part of the food tracker is that it helps you to be aware of how many calories you're consuming day-to-day, and what foods those calories are coming from.

The food glossary helps you to identify your favorite foods so that you can be more aware of your eating habits. When you can identify those patterns you can modify them as needed should you choose to do so. You have been tracking your food intake for a week now, so you should start seeing some patterns emerge.

Don't worry about modifying your food intake just yet. We're not going to start doing that until you've been tracking your food for four weeks. This four-week period is establishing a baseline of what your eating habits are so that you can determine what to change and how to change it if needed.

KEY POINTS TO REMEMBER FOR LESSON 2

- The only way change happens is when the pain of staying the same is higher than the pain of changing.

- Your Statement of Purpose and Change Plan are at the heart of the Natural Eating program. Without both of these documents, the chances of success are greatly decreased

- The Statement of Purpose is the "what," what you're trying to accomplish, and the Change Plan is the "how," how you plan to accomplish it.

- Don't make any major changes on your eating habits yet. Instead, use the Food Tracker to establish a baseline of your eating habits.

LESSON 3

INTUITIVE EATING AND MINDFUL EATING

As we mentioned in Lesson 1, the Natural Eating Program has two major components. Those components are *Intuitive Eating* and *Mindful Eating*.

In this Lesson we'll be discussing *Intuitive Eating*.

The information below comes from the website, The *Original Intuitive Eating Pros* found at https://www.intuitiveeating.org/

There are ten major principles of Intuitive Eating. As you read over these points, consider your own relationship with food and how integrating these ten principles might help you begin to change your relationship with food and with eating.

As you fill out your Food Tracker for this week, pay particular attention to how the principles below impact your food choices. Don't worry about changing anything yet, just be mindful of how your eating habits might be reflected in the principles of Intuitive Eating outlined below.

1. Reject the Diet Mentality

The diet industry has a vested interest in failure. If their diets worked, then you wouldn't need to keep going back to the well to buy more of their books, videos, and programs to help you lose weight.

Remember the only rule of weight loss from Lesson 1: Consume less calories than you burn. It's really that simple, but almost impossible to actually do. That's because we've been lied to by the diet industry that if we just find the "right" diet or eat the "right" foods we'll finally be able to lose weight successfully.

2. Honor Your Hunger

Most people say "hunger" when they mean "appetite." While appetite is merely the desire or the craving for a food, hunger is an actual physical sensation.

Hunger manifests in stomach rumbles or the feeling of an empty stomach. It may also show up as a feeling of depleted energy or tiredness during the day.

Appetite, on the other hand, is just the desire to eat, absent any of the symptoms of hunger. People usually indulge their appetites by eating when they're bored or out of sorts emotionally.

You can honor your hunger by only eating when you're hungry, and by stopping when you're satisfied (as opposed to full). How do you know when you're satisfied?

We'll talk about that more in the next Lesson when we discuss Mindful Eating, but for now let's just say that when you feel yourself losing interest in what you are eating, or when your craving or hunger are gone, you are satisfied.

3. Make Peace with Food

The way to make peace with food is to give yourself unconditional permission to eat. Unless you have to avoid certain foods out of medical necessity, no food is off the table.

If you want chocolate, have chocolate. If you want pizza, have pizza. If you want ice cream, eat some ice cream. When you honor your hunger by stopping when you're satisfied instead of eating until you're full, you come to realize that what's important is the quality of the food and not the quantity.

Do two bites of ice cream really taste better than one bite of ice cream? What if you could enjoy one bite of ice cream twice as much? Could you then cut your ice cream consumption in half?

If you tell yourself that you can't or shouldn't have certain foods, you'll feel guilty when you do eat them. If you're an emotional eater, guilt is an emotion.

Feeling guilty is what leads to binge-eating for emotional eaters. If certain foods are off the list, and then you finally give in to cravings for those foods, the guilt takes over. This can lead to even more guilt and more binge eating until you reach "f-it" mode. At that point, you're thinking things like, "This is hopeless; I can't do this, so I might as well enjoy myself."

Once you have reached this stage of eating, you're overwhelmed with guilt after the binge, and the cycle starts all over again. You can make peace with food by remembering that the quantity of your favorite snacks is not as important as the quality of the experience of eating them.

4. Challenge the Food Police

The classic and most universal example of the food police comes from a childhood where one or both parents told you to "clean your plate" before you could leave the table. In reality, you should leave the table when you feel satisfied. It's okay to leave food on your plate. You can save it for tomorrow.

Get rid of the idea that you're "bad" because you didn't clean your plate, or because you ate a piece of chocolate cake. Say "no" to that voice in your head that tells you that you are "good" because you ate a salad or cleaned your plate.

Food is what it is. Unless you have food allergies or other medical conditions that prevent you from eating certain foods, learn to let go of the "food cop" who lives in your head. If you place judgments on yourself for feeling guilty or "bad" about eating certain foods, then that can start the guilt/binge cycle all over again, leading to even more guilt-induced bingeing.

Another challenge the food police try to brainwash you with is that you have to eat certain foods at certain times of the day. Let go of the "rules" that you have to eat breakfast by 9 a.m., lunch at noon, and dinner by 6 p.m.

Natural eating means listening to what your body tells you, and not what the food police think should be your eating schedule. Eat when you are hungry, stop when you are satisfied, and tell the food police to get lost.

5. Discover the Satisfaction Factor

Does this experience sound familiar? You want a piece of chocolate, but you've been conditioned by the food police to believe that chocolate is bad for you, so you choose to snack on something "healthy" instead.

You eat a cup of grapes, but find after eating them that your craving for chocolate is still there, so you eat some whole grain avocado toast, only to find that the craving is still there. So you continue eating "healthy" alternatives to chocolate only to find that none of them satisfy your craving for chocolate.

The reason for this should be obvious: Only chocolate can satisfy a craving for chocolate. You won't feel satisfied until you actually eat some chocolate.

Note that "some" chocolate doesn't mean ALL of the chocolate. You can satisfy your craving for chocolate without eating a whole bar or a whole bag. The reason for this is that two bites of chocolate are not any more delicious than one bite of chocolate.

If you learn to savor every bite, then you can learn to be satisfied with fewer bites. There will be an exercise in next week's Lesson that will go into more depth on how to do this, but for now here's something to experiment with. After every bite of your favorite food, pause, put down your fork (or spoon) and ask yourself, "Am I satisfied yet?"

This act of slowing down and consciously enjoying your food will help you to discover your own satisfaction factor and to learn to be more satisfied with less food.

6. Feel Your Fullness

If you learn to ignore the food police and to trust your own body, it will tell you when you are satisfied. In future Lesson s we're going to say more about how to listen to what your body tells you so that you can leave the table satisfied but not stuffed.

For now, just practice listening to what your body is telling you while you are eating. Make eating a conscious act by not doing anything else while eating. Focus all of your attention on the experience of eating, paying particular attention to how your body responds to food.

Slow down and enjoy every morsel, giving your body time to let you know when it has been satisfied.

7. Cope with Your Emotions with Kindness

Most of us associate food with comfort. In most cultures food means family, celebration, and pleasant times spent together. It's no wonder that we have learned to soothe our emotions through food. Unfortunately, food doesn't fix feelings. It only takes our minds off of them temporarily.

Sadness, fear, anxiety, loneliness, boredom, and anger are all emotions that everyone experiences from time to time. Food won't fix any of these feelings.

Food can only act as a distraction that prevents us from dealing with the root of the emotion. How do you know if you are engaging in emotional eating?

Think about the word "HALT." If you are tempted to eat because you feel Helpless, Angry, Lonely or Tired, you are engaging in emotional eating. Before you eat anything, first ask yourself if you're eating because you're hungry, or if you're eating because of "HALT."

If you feel tempted to eat when you're not hungry, then treat yourself with kindness instead. Ask yourself what the root of the feeling is, and then ask yourself how you can deal with it in a kind and loving way.

Sometimes the only way to deal with it is just to sit quietly with it and allow yourself to experience it without having to react to it, in a mindful manner. When you are able to do this you will have the key to stop emotional eating.

8. Respect Your Body

I'd love to be tall enough to play basketball in the professional leagues. Unfortunately I was born too short for that. I'd also love to be one of those people who can eat as much as they want of whatever they want without gaining weight, but my genetic blueprint had other plans for me.

One of the great things about the human race is that we're all born different sizes, shapes, and colors. This diversity is our true beauty. If everyone looked exactly the same, imagine how boring that would be.

If you have unrealistic expectations about changing your body size or shape, it'll be nearly impossible to reject the diet mentality. In extreme cases it can lead to eating disorders. Like you, your body is unique and deserves dignity and respect. Appreciate you for who you are and you'll be well on your way to eating naturally.

9. Movement—Feel the Difference

It's a common myth that if you exercise regularly you can lose weight. The average candy bar is 200 calories. To burn that off, you'd have to do 30 minutes of cardio-intensive aerobic exercise or an hour of moderate calisthenics or weight lifting.

That doesn't mean you shouldn't exercise though. It means you should change your reasons and motivations for exercise. Do it for the way it makes you feel. Exercise stimulates beta endorphins, which are the body's natural antidepressants. Exercise also reduces the body's stress-producing hormone, cortisol. If you get moving you'll feel better about yourself, which will reduce the tendency towards emotional eating.

If you exercise because it makes you feel good instead of because it burns calories, you'll come to realize that any physical activity is good.

With this knowledge comes the realization that the type of activity doesn't matter as long as you're moving, so you can indulge yourself by doing things you enjoy instead of plodding off to the gym every day. Go for a swim. Ride a mountain bike. Or just take a short walk in the park or around the neighborhood.

What's important is not so much the type of movement as to get moving in the first place.

If you have difficulty encouraging yourself to exercise, try the Two-Minute Rule. Instead of telling yourself, "I need to exercise for an hour today," just tell yourself you'll exercise for two minutes. Then at the end of two minutes, see if you'd like to keep moving.

The hard part of exercise for most people is to get moving in the first place. The Two-Minute Rule helps you to get over that first hurdle. Usually once you actually get moving, it's easy to keep going. And even if it isn't, you can always quit after two minutes and try again tomorrow.

The Exercise Police are just as nefarious as the Food Police. When you learn to say "no" to both, you'll be free to exercise on your own time table by listening to your own body.

10. Honor Your Health—Gentle Nutrition

One of the reasons you're currently tracking your food intake is that it helps you to identify your likes and dislikes and to make informed decisions about the nutritional content of your food. You don't have to eat "perfectly" all the time. You can honor your health while still eating the foods that make you feel good and that satisfy you. One bite or one meal that isn't "perfect" isn't going to suddenly make you unhealthy. Unhealthy foods eaten over long periods of time, or habitually, are what cause ill health and obesity. You can occasionally indulge as long as you don't make indulging a daily habit.

The information in your Food Tracker will help you to identify which foods you enjoy are most healthy, and which are least healthy. You can then use that information to make informed natural eating choices by eating more of what's healthy and less of what's not healthy.

This doesn't mean you have to eliminate the "unhealthy" foods altogether. It just means being aware of what they are so you can practice mindful eating with them, focusing on the satisfaction factor, so you can be more satisfied with a smaller quantity of those foods.

By tracking your food you will also learn what healthy foods are the most satisfying to you so that you can eat them more consistently over longer periods of time. You don't have to be "perfect" in your food choices as long as you make progress in changing your relationship with food.

Remember that the only rule is to eat less than you burn. One way to do this is to honor your health through gently making more healthy food choices while realizing you don't have to completely give up your favorite snacks.

FOOD TRACKER

Look at the "quantity" (serving size) column on your food tracker. See if you can identify which foods you eat the most of in terms of quantity. Now look at the nutrition information for that food. What's the calorie content? The protein content? The fat content? The carbohydrate content? The sugar content? Is this food "healthy" or "unhealthy" for you based on your evaluation of this information?

If it's a "healthy" food, could you increase your intake of it? If it's an "unhealthy" food, could you train yourself to be more satisfied with a smaller quantity of it by focusing on the satisfaction factor as outlined in item #5 from the list above?

This information can always be used to modify the foods you eat so that you are eating more "healthy" foods and less "unhealthy" foods without feeling that you have to completely give up certain foods.

KEY POINTS TO REMEMBER FOR LESSON 3

- Learn to distinguish between "hunger" and "appetite." Hunger is a physical sensation; appetite is simply the desire to eat.

- Stop eating when you are satisfied, not when you are full.

- Only restrict certain foods is for medical reasons. Otherwise, eat what you want, in smaller portions.

- Quality, not quantity, is what's important in satisfying your food cravings.

- Stop emotional eating by thinking "HALT:" Never eat when you feel Helpless, Angry, Lonely, or Tired.

- Use your food tracker to increase the amount of healthy foods you eat while decreasing the unhealthy foods you eat.

- Decreasing unhealthy foods doesn't mean eliminating them altogether. You can still enjoy your favorite foods if you learn to be more satisfied with smaller quantities.

REFERENCES

10 Principles of Intuitive Eating
Reprinted with permission from:
Tribole E and Resch E. Intuitive Eating, 2nd ed. (1995, 2003), NY:NY.
www.IntuitiveEating.org

Cadena-Schlam, Leslie and López-Guimerà, Gemma 2015). *Intuitive eating: An emerging approach to eating behavior*, Department of Clinical and Health Psychology. Universitat Autònoma de Barcelona. Barcelona. Spain.

Van Dyke, Nina and Drinkwater, Eric J. (2013). Relationships between intuitive eating and health indicators: literature review, *Public Health Nutrition, August 2013*.

LESSON 4

MINDFUL EATING

How often do you find yourself doing other things while eating? How often do you sit down, relax, and take time to enjoy your food?

Mindful Eating is about being present in the moment with your meal so that you may fully enjoy it and be more satisfied with it. Mindful Eating also helps you to listen to your body's signals so you will know whether you are hungry or just have an appetite.

One aspect of changing your relationship with food is to move from Doing Mode into Being Mode. In Doing Mode we're trying to accomplish things. Eating in Doing Mode means focusing on ending the process of eating as quickly as possible to get on to the next thing on the day's agenda.

Being Mode with eating means just being with the process of eating so that we may savor each bite of the meal.

The six skills outlined below are designed to move you from Doing Mode to Being Mode when eating.

In Doing Mode we're trying to "fix" things or check off items on our agendas. We may be stuck inside our heads, thinking about endless "to do" lists or focusing on things other than the present activity we're engaged in.

Doing Mode leads to unconscious, mindless eating habits. If you've ever caught yourself eating without being aware of it, or if you've ever polished off a whole bag of chips when you only meant to eat a few, you were probably engaged in Doing Mode at the time.

Being Mode, on the other hand, is moving away from thinking and doing to just being in the present moment with an activity. In Mindful Eating, Being Mode is the act of allowing yourself to be present with your food, enjoying every morsel.

In essence, Mindful Eating allows you to do just that: Shift from Doing Mode to Being Mode.

The "What" and "How" Skills of Mindful Eating

(from a concept by Marsha Linehan, founder of Dialectical Behavior Therapy)

There are six skills of Mindful Eating. These skills are designed to allow you to shift from Doing Mode to Being Mode and to be fully present with the experience of eating. In Being Mode you are more readily able to pinpoint the exact moment when you are satisfied so you can stop eating at that point.

The skills of Mindful Eating are divided up into "what" skills and "how" skills. The "what" skills are what you do to be mindful, and the "how" skills are how you do it.

The "What" Skills of Mindful Eating (what to do to eat mindfully) are:

Observing

When we are preoccupied with thoughts of the past or the future, we are in thinking mode. Thinking mode takes us away from experiencing the world directly with our senses; or sensing mode. Mindful Awareness teaches us to focus on the world experienced directly by our senses: touch, taste, smell, hearing, and sight. Experiencing life in sensing mode introduces us to a richer world. It's impossible to be bored or apathetic if you treat each experience as if it is happening to you for the first time, through your senses. Mindful eating helps you to have sensory experiences in the present. When you use the skill of observing while engaging in mindful eating, you are focusing all of your senses on the experience of eating. We're all accustomed to using our sense of taste to enjoy a meal, but how might you engage your other senses as well? Could you take a moment prior to eating the meal to appreciate the way it is presented on the plate? To enjoy the colors and aromas of the food? To feel the textures on your tongue? To hear the pleasant crunching sounds of a crisp piece of fruit? The more you can observe the meal through your senses, the more you will increase your enjoyment of the experience.

Describing

This skill of Mindful Eating involves observing the smallest details of the meal, then putting the experience into words. Describing means approaching each meal as if you are experiencing it for the first time. Explore as many dimensions of it as you can, then describe it to yourself. You already know what your meal tastes like, but what does it smell like? What does it look like? What does it sound like? What does it feel like? When you engage your mindful powers of describing you increase your satisfaction of the meal.

Participating

Mindful Eating allows you to experience every aspect of your food. As you engage in Mindful Eating, set aside any other activities. Turn off the television. Shut down the smart phone. Set aside the books and magazines and allow yourself to truly and fully enjoy the meal by participating in it. If necessary, set your fork or spoon down after every bite so that you can savor it before going on to the next one. See if you can pinpoint the exact moment when your food has satisfied you and you no longer have to continue eating.

The "How" Skills of Mindful Eating (how to eat mindfully) are:

Being Non-judgmental

Mindful Eating teaches us the art of acceptance. Being non-judgmental means seeing the world as it is, without judgments or assumptions. When we can do so, we have achieved Beginner's Mind or Child's Mind, which is the art of experiencing everything as if seeing it for the first time.

Being non-judgmental in Mindful Eating means not labeling your food or your eating habits as "good" or "bad," but instead linking choices to consequences in a positive, intentional way without blaming, shaming or guilt-tripping yourself or others over your food choices.

Being One-Mindful

Being one-mindful just means focusing on one thing at a time.

The journey of a thousand miles begins with a single step. If we focus on the final destination at the end of a thousand miles, we'll get so overwhelmed with the task at hand that we may be afraid to even take the first step.

But if we ask ourselves, "what is the smallest thing I can do today to make a difference?" and then just focus on that one thing before going on to the next, we're mindfully using all of our attention to be present in the moment.

If there's any energy left over after doing that one thing, we can then go on to the next, and then the next, until the task is complete.

Because of our busy lives, when we're eating we often add sitting down to a meal to our checklist of things to accomplish during the day. When we look at eating in that manner we tend to rush through the meal, not even taking time to savor and enjoy the experience.

But if we can learn to slow down and be in the moment with our food we can get more enjoyment out of it, and be more satisfied with less food.

The Last Kiss activity at the end of this week's lesson is an exercise in being present in the moment with our food. When you try this activity, notice how it changes the way you approach eating.

Does it feel more natural to eat in this manner?

Being Intentional

This is probably the most important skill of Mindful Eating, because it teaches us to focus on solutions, not problems. We can talk about problems all day, but until we start talking about solutions, nothing will ever get solved. The way to solve a problem is to take positive, intentional steps towards finding a solution.

All of the skills of Mindful Eating come together in the power of intention.

A mindful life is a life lived deliberately. Such a consciously lived life is not driven about on the winds of whim and fortune. It is a purposeful life.

The power of intention helps us to solve problems in a purposeful manner. It is possible to live a life of purpose through tapping into this power. The way to use the power of intention is to begin by asking two questions:

1. What am I trying to accomplish here?

2. Are my thoughts, feelings, and behaviors going to help me to achieve this goal?

When we live in mindful awareness, our thoughts, behaviors, and actions always support our intention. When you practice Mindful Eating, you are engaging in a solution-focused, effective way to change your relationship with food without guilt, shame or blame.

Mindful Eating: The Last Kiss

I love chocolate. There have been times when I've been absent-mindedly eating chocolate kisses while working on the computer.

On occasion when I'm doing this I've reached into the bag only to find it empty. At those times I've thought to myself, "I wish I'd realized that the last one I ate was the last kiss in the bag! If I had known, I would have paid more attention to it!"

There was nothing different about the last kiss in the bag. It was just like all the other kisses in the bag. What was different was the fact that I should have been focusing my attention on it.

What if we were able to focus our attention on every kiss in the bag? What if we could make every kiss as important as the last one?

Try the exercise below with a piece of chocolate. If you cannot eat chocolate, or if you just don't like chocolate, you may wish to use a raisin or other small food item. Make it a bite-sized food item that you really enjoy eating.

When you are ready with the food item, try the exercise outlined below.

- Hold the chocolate in your hand. Don't unwrap it or put it in your mouth yet. Simply observe it and describe it to yourself as you hold it in your hand. Picture yourself as an artist about to draw this piece of chocolate. How many colors do you see? What is its shape? How do the light and the shadow fall on it? If you were going to draw it, how would you go about doing so?

- Now unwrap the chocolate and hold the wrapper up to your ear. Close your eyes and rub the wrapper between your fingers. What does it sound like? If you were a blind person, would you be able to identify the wrapper simply by the sound it makes?

- Explore the food item with your other senses before putting it in your mouth. How does it feel in your hand? What is its texture. Smell it. Could you identify it solely from the smell?

- Now place the chocolate on your tongue, but don't bite it. Allow it to slowly dissolve.

- Where on your tongue can you first taste it? On the front of your tongue, on the back of your tongue, or somewhere in the middle?

- The four basic taste buds are sweet, sour, salt and bitter. Can you taste each of these sensations? Which one did you taste first?

- Pay close attention to your sense of smell. Can you notice any aroma as you eat the chocolate?

- Now savor the chocolate as if it is the last piece of chocolate on earth. If this were the last piece of chocolate on earth, and you were aware that this would be the last time you could ever taste chocolate, how would it change your experience of the sensation of eating it?

- Before chewing and swallowing, allow yourself to move from Doing Mode to Being Mode with the eating experience.

- Enjoy and savor the moment with this bit of food. There is nothing to do right now but to experience this piece of chocolate.

- When you are ready, begin to chew the chocolate, savoring every flavor as you do so. Continue to be present in the moment with the chocolate, allowing yourself to fully participate in the experience, until you are done.

When engaging in Mindful Eating, be in the moment with the experience. Being one-mindful in Mindful Eating means realizing that you have nowhere to go and nothing to do but to enjoy the experience of eating here and now, in this moment.

Did the exercise above change your experience of chocolate in any way? If so, you've learned the art of fully participating in Mindful Eating.

FOOD TRACKER

You've been tracking your food for four weeks now, so you should have a good baseline to start modifying your food intake naturally. For the remainder of the lessons in this program we're going to be looking at how to do that.

Remember that the only rule of weight loss is to burn more than you consume, or to consume less than you burn.

Take another look at your Food Tracker and pay particular attention to the "calories" column. Where do you seem to be getting most of your calories?

Now look at the "Satisfaction" column and relate it to the "calories" column. Is there a relationship between the amount of calories and the level of satisfaction for the foods on your list?

Now pick a few of your highest calorie items on the list. If you eat them again in the following week, practice Mindful Eating this time as you do.

Did the amount of food you ate change when you ate mindfully?

POINTS TO REMEMBER FOR LESSON 4

- The way to eat mindfully is to shift from Doing Mode to Being Mode while eating.

- Mindful Eating consists of three "what" skills and three "how" skills

- The "what" skills are what you do to eat mindfully, and the "how" skills are how you do it

- The "what" skills are:
    - o Observing
    - o Describing

o Participating

- The "how" skills are:
    o Being Non-judgmental
    o Being One-mindful
    o Being Intentional (Effective)

REFERENCES

Linehan, Marsha & Wilks, Chelsey. (2015). The Course and Evolution of
    Dialectical Behavior Therapy. *American journal of psychotherapy*. 69. 97-
    110. 10.1176/appi.psychotherapy.2015.69.2.97.

Lofgren, Ingrid. (2015). Mindful Eating. *American Journal of Lifestyle Medicine*.
    9. 10.1177/1559827615569684.

LESSON 5

CEASE THE DIET MENTALITY

Dieting involves restricting yourself to eating certain kinds of foods while avoiding certain other kinds. Dieting often induces feelings of guilt when people cannot avoid certain foods. This guilt often leads to emotional eating, which induces more guilt, which leads to more emotional eating.

It's a vicious cycle and the chief reason why most diets fail.

Natural eating, on the other hand, doesn't mean restricting or eliminating certain kinds of foods. With natural eating, unless you have a medical reason for avoiding certain foods, no food is off the table.

The only rule to losing weight is to consume less than you burn. Natural eating isn't about restricting the types of food you eat. It's about becoming aware of how you eat, and respecting your body's signals regarding your food intake.

At any given time in America, at least 45 million Americans are on a diet. In spite of this, studies by the Centers for Disease Control estimate that 42% of Americans are overweight.

If diets work, why is America an obese nation? Why is the number of overweight Americans increasing instead of decreasing?

Diets Don't Work

While many people who diet can lose up to 10% of their body weight in the short term, research demonstrates that most gain it back over the long term. According to a UCLA study, many even gain back more weight than they initially lost!

Part of the reason for this is that diets are temporary solutions to a permanent problem. We restrict certain foods long enough to lose weight, but once the weight is lost we go back to our old eating habits, and the weight returns.

Not only that, but dieting doesn't change the way we think about food in the long term. It can lead to obsessive thoughts about the kinds of food you can eat when the diet is over, and since diets don't satisfy our natural cravings for certain types of foods, it can lead to binge eating. And binge eating triggers the guilt cycle all over again.

Diets also slow the metabolism, which means that if you go back to your normal way of eating after the diet is over, without making permanent lifestyle changes, you will gain more weight with eating the same amounts of food. This is because you're now not burning the food as fast as you were prior to the diet.

Our bodies naturally react to food deprivation by going into "famine" mode. Our metabolism slows, and we start storing more nutrients. This state is known as "homeostasis."

Dieting or fasting triggers the body to go into starvation mode, because our biological processes react to food deprivation by storing more energy than usual in the form of fat. Our bodies have a natural tendency to try to restore balance when changes are made, and dieting works against these natural biological processes.

Ceasing the Diet Mentality

Dieting is a temporary solution to a permanent problem. Dieting attempts to reduce weight over a short period of time. This doesn't work because for the rest of your life you will have to eat to live, and if the changes you make aren't permanent, they'll return when you are no longer dieting.

Change can be difficult if you have been conditioned to believing that maintaining a healthy weight is solely a matter of depriving yourself of foods you truly love or believing that there are short-term solutions that can fix lifelong eating patterns.

Part of the diet mentality is the belief that when diets fail, it's the fault of the dieter instead of the diet; however, if that were true, then the majority of dieting Americans wouldn't keep gaining weight.

If, on the other hand, you are willing to commit to making permanent changes while rejecting the idea that you have to deprive yourself of certain foods, you can learn to eat naturally and maintain a healthy weight.

When you have learned to do so by using the techniques in the Natural Eating Program, you will have permanently changed your relationship with food so that you can have a healthy lifestyle for the rest of your life.

The diet mentality makes the assumption that Body-Mass Index (BMI) is the sole factor in determining health, but recent research demonstrates that this may not be the case.

A 2012 study by the Journal of the American Board of Family Medicine found that a lifestyle that includes eating 5 or more fruits and vegetables daily, exercising regularly, consuming alcohol in moderation, and not smoking are associated with a significant decrease in mortality regardless of baseline BMI.

Natural Eating recognizes that adopting healthy lifestyle habits is more important than simply being thinner for the sake of being thin. Dieting can actually be harmful if it deprives the body of needed nutrients in the quest for weight loss. In extreme cases it can lead to eating disorders like Anorexia and Bulimia.

You don't have to be thin to be healthy. If you adopt the lifestyle changes mentioned above you can decrease your risk of serious illnesses while maintaining permanent lifestyle changes.

Another component of the diet mindset is that you have to be thin to be attractive. This is a product of culture more than of science. Although this idea is being challenged in recent years, I'm sure we've all seen photographs of runway models who are bordering on anorexic.

Dr. Adrienne Key, a psychiatrist who works with eating disorders, estimates that about 20% to 40% of fashion models are currently experiencing an eating disorder. Sacrificing your health on the altar of being fashionable is obviously not a sustainable lifestyle, and in many instances it can be dangerous if not deadly.

Bodies come in all shapes and sizes. Part of rejecting the diet mentality is learning to be happy in your own skin, regardless of your current BMI. Ironically, this knowledge alone is often enough to make losing weight easier, because it eliminates the pressure, and therefore the stress, of dieting.

Benefits of Ceasing the Diet Mentality

If you've ever been on a diet, I'm sure you're familiar with the fact that when you're dieting you're constantly obsessing over food and thinking about what you can eat next.

Nothing makes a thing more attractive than telling yourself you can't have it. So the more we think about what we can eat next, the more we obsess over it. Obsessing over food is exactly what leads to binge eating.

When you stop dieting you stop obsessing over food, because there's no food you cannot eat if you're not on a diet.

Another thing that happens when you cease the diet mentality is that your craving for sweets and carbohydrates decreases.

You may have noticed that on your Food Tracker one of the things you're tracking is the carbohydrate content of the foods you're eating. This isn't because you're trying to restrict the amount of carbohydrates you intake on a daily basis (unless there's a medical reason for doing so).

Instead, you're gathering that information to be aware of your daily, weekly, and monthly carbohydrate intake to see if and how it changes over time.

Carbohydrates are energy. When your body goes into starvation mode (which happens frequently with diets) it acts to try to correct the situation. Carbohydrates are your body's instant energy resource.

If your body feels it is being deprived, it will naturally seek quick energy in the form of carbohydrates and sugars.

When you cease the diet mentality you give yourself permission to eat whatever you want whenever you want it. The more you try to restrict your carbohydrate and sugar intake, the more your body craves it.

But if you give yourself permission to have a slice of cake or a piece of chocolate once in a while, your body isn't going into starvation mode, so you naturally crave less carbohydrates and sugars.

You may notice that when you give yourself permission to enjoy carbohydrates from time to time, your hunger will naturally shift to healthier carbohydrates like whole grains and high fiber vegetables and fruits instead of cookies, cakes, and candy. This is because you haven't upset your body's natural balance through dieting.

When you cease the diet mentality you will also become more proficient at recognizing your body's hunger and satisfaction cues. It you're like most people, when you're dieting your thoughts are constantly on the next meal.

Let's do a thought experiment. Suppose for a day or two you gave yourself permission to eat whatever you wanted, whenever you wanted it. You sit down at the table with a gallon of ice cream, a cake, some pies, a big basket of chocolates, and whatever other indulgences you've been denying yourself all this time, and start eating.

How long do you think it would be before you said to yourself, "Alright, I've had enough!" If you're not dieting, how would you know when it's time to stop eating?

The answer, of course, is that you would have to listen to your body telling you that it was satisfied. Dieting means you are rarely if ever satisfied. Ceasing the diet mentality means you're learning to let your body tell you when it's satisfied.

Another benefit of ceasing the diet mentality is that you can stop eating when you are satisfied.

This means that you don't have to "clean your plate" because if you're hungry again in an hour you can eat again in an hour. Instead of trying to force your body into an arbitrary "three meals a day" schedule, you eat more naturally by eating when you're hungry and stopping when you're satisfied.

Ceasing the Guilt

When you let go of the diet mentality, you exercise your mindful skill of being non-judgmental by letting go of the idea that certain foods are "good" and certain foods are "bad." If you can eat whatever you want whenever you want, you tend to only eat when you actually want something.

In other words, you respond to your hunger instead of to your appetite. When you do this, you eliminate feeling guilty about eating. As we've already discussed multiple times, binge-eating is usually the result of guilt. You eat one of the "forbidden" foods, which leads to feelings of guilt, which leads to eating even more, which eventually results in bingeing.

When you cease the guilt, you cease the bingeing that can result from it.

A final benefit of ceasing the diet mentality is that you will find that your weight will probably stabilize. Forbidding or restricting certain foods leads to "yo-yo dieting," where you repeatedly lose weight only to gain it back when the diet is over.

If you don't forbid yourself to eat certain foods, you cease the diet mentality, and therefore the yo-yo dieting. You may even find that your weight stabilizes at a lower BMI than you were able to achieve through dieting, because you are no longer subjecting your body to endless cycles of deprivation followed by weight gain.

FOOD TRACKER

On your Food Tracker this week, pay particular attention to the columns marked "carbohydrates" and "sugar." Compare the daily carbohydrate and sugar counts starting with the first day you tracked them to now. Did you notice any change over time? Are you able to spot any trends or patterns?

Now look at the column marked "protein." Protein is the stuff that satisfies your sense of being full. The more protein per calorie of intake, the more satisfied you feel. Did you notice any trends there? How does it relate to your carbohydrate and sugar intake?

POINTS TO REMEMBER FOR LESSON 5

- Natural eating means ceasing the diet mentality by letting go of the idea that there are "good" foods and "bad" foods.

- When you stop trying to eliminate certain foods, you naturally learn to be more in tune with your body's natural senses of hunger and satisfaction.

- Diets don't work because they're a temporary solution to a permanent problem.

- Thin doesn't necessarily mean healthy. There's less relationship between BMI and health than between positive lifestyle choices and health.

- Let go of binge eating by letting go of the guilt induced by the diet mentality.

REFERENCES

Mann, T., Tomiyama, A., Westling, E., Lew, A., Samuels, B., & Chatman, J. (2007). Medicare's search for effective obesity treatments: diets are not

the answer. *The American psychologist,* 62(3), 220-233.
http://dx.doi.org/10.1037/0003-066x.62.3.220 Retrieved from
https://escholarship.org/uc/item/2811g3r3

Matheson, Eric M., King, Dana E. and Everett, Charles J. (2012). Healthy
Lifestyle Habits and Mortality in Overweight and Obese Individuals,
Journal of the American Board of Family Medicine: first published as
10.3122/jabfm.2012.01.110164 on 4 January 2012.
Downloaded from http://www.jabfm.org/ on September 14, 2021.

LESSON 6

CONSCIOUS EATING

Most of the time when we have problems with our food intake it's because we practice unconscious eating.

How often have you found yourself eating without even being aware of it?

How often have you set out to eat a small portion of something then found yourself eating a lot more than you intended?

How often have you found yourself eating when you weren't hungry?

How often have you experienced "Thanksgiving Syndrome," where you eat so much that you're uncomfortable afterwards?

If you've experienced any of these things, you've experienced unconscious eating.

Natural Eating involves becoming consciously aware of what you're eating and when. When you have mastered the art of eating consciously, you'll be able to do all of these things:

Eat slowly, without distractions, savoring and enjoying every morsel of food

Listen to your body's cues so that you will know when you are satisfied

- Be able to stop eating when you're satisfied without feeling stuffed
- Know the difference between hunger and appetite
- Activate your satisfaction cues by noticing the colors, smells, textures, sounds, flavors, and the overall experience of enjoying your food
- Cope with emotions without resorting to food
- Eat to maintain your physical and emotional health and not to satisfy your appetite
- Become aware of the effects what you eat has on your mood, your energy levels, and your overall sense of wellbeing
- Appreciate your food more
- Know when to stop eating
- Replace automatic, unconscious thought processes about food and eating with conscious, intentional and intuitive eating habits

On the other hand, unconscious, mindless eating involves the following:

- Distracted eating or eating while bored
- Not paying attention to what or why you're eating
- Ignoring your body's cues when it's telling you that you've had enough
- Eating out of boredom, craving, or emotional cues instead of because you're hungry
- Ignoring your body's satisfaction cues
- Eating to satisfy your appetite while ignoring your physical and emotional health
- Not paying attention to how your mood, energy levels and overall sense of wellbeing effects your appetite
- Never feeling satisfied with your food
- Not being able to stop eating
- Engaging in unconscious, mindless eating

This week, any time you eat something, notice what the experience is like for you. Do you do any of the things listed above?

If you find yourself eating without being aware of it, stop what you're doing and review the two lists above. If you're still feeling hungry afterwards, go ahead and continue eating; but if you're not, listen to what your body is telling you and wait to eat when you are hungry and not because you're trying to satisfy your appetite.

Hunger vs. Appetite

As mentioned in previous lessons, there is a difference between hunger and appetite. Most, if not all, unconscious eating occurs as a result of trying to satisfy your appetite instead of trying to satisfy your hunger.

So how do you know the difference between hunger and appetite? The chart on the next page explains the differences.

HUNGER	**APPETITE**
A physical sensation	The desire to eat something
In the body	In the mind
Need	Want (craving)
Need for fuel (leading to lack of physical energy)	Want something to do (boredom, emotional triggers)
Will eat almost anything	Eating specific foods
Gradual	Sudden
No mental trigger (no prior mental or emotional cues)	Mental trigger (boredom, craving, emotional triggers, emotional comfort-seeking)
Mindful	Mindless
Intuitive	Not intuitive

Some additional signs of hunger include difficulty concentrating, loss of energy, feeling faint or light-headed, headaches, increased irritability, and a mild rumbling in the stomach.

To practice Conscious Eating, the next time you find yourself about to eat something, first ask yourself, "Am I really hungry, or do I just have an appetite for something?"

If you're just eating because of appetite, wait until you're truly hungry and find something else to do.

Alternately, you can switch from Doing Mode to Being Mode and just sit with the craving until it goes away.

Ride the Wave

We're all familiar with substance abuse and addictive behaviors. When a person has a substance abuse problem, they mindlessly engage in partaking of substances that are detrimental to their health.

Did you know that it's also possible to become addicted to a process? Process addictions occur when we find ourselves engaging in behaviors that can be harmful to our health.

Unconscious eating can be a type of process addiction because it is a result of trying to satisfy a craving or an appetite rather than eating to satisfy your body's needs. Too much unconscious eating is obviously bad for your health.

Our bodies are complex systems of cycles. These cycles peak and trough throughout the day, and throughout our lifetimes. They come and go in waves.

When certain waves peak together, that's when those cravings hit. We may crave sugar, or chocolate, or other types of food with lower nutritional value. When we're on top of that wave, it can feel like that urge is never going to go away.

But since these changes occur in cycles, if you can "ride the wave," those urges will eventually subside. If we don't give in to them, and wait patiently for them to go away, we can take conscious, intentional control of our eating habits.

Conscious eating helps us to know our bodies and their complex cycles. It also helps us to know that "this too shall pass."

If you are troubled by unconscious eating habits, the way to "ride the wave" is to shift from Doing Mode to Being Mode, sitting quietly in the moment with the craving to indulge. We all know from our personal experiences with food that the craving will eventually subside. this is true even though it may feel in the moment as if the craving is never going to go away.

If we are able, just for a moment, to let go of the urge to indulge, then another moment, then another, eventually the craving or appetite will subside.

Even if it doesn't, mindful awareness gives us the knowledge that we are not our cravings. We are in control, if we choose to be. And we can mindfully choose to observe and describe the cravings to ourselves without having to act upon them.

The more practice we have at this, the more we will be able to let go of those craving cycles when they occur. With practice riding the wave, we can move from unconscious eating to conscious eating.

Beat the Clock

We've been conditioned to "eat three square meals a day." That's great if your meal schedule matches your hunger schedule, but what if it's meal time and you're not hungry? Should you force yourself to eat out of some arbitrary habit?

Most people need to eat something every four or five hours to give the body sufficient fuel to go about daily business, but every human body is different and we all have different metabolic rates. Just because I may feel hungry every five hours, that doesn't mean that you will be on the same schedule.

When you begin to practice conscious eating, you will intuitively learn your body's natural hunger cycles. You may be surprised to learn that your hunger cycles don't match up with "meal time."

If that's the case, be prepared to listen to what your body is telling you instead of what the clock is telling you, and eat accordingly.

You may also find that as you begin to practice conscious eating you may require four or five smaller meals throughout the day instead of three bigger meals. This eating style, commonly referred to as "grazing," began as a fad in the 1980s.

If you are "grazing" because it's what your body is telling you to do, that's fine, but don't get caught up in the idea that mini-meals are always the correct solution for everybody. The correct eating cycle for you is the one that your body tells you to follow.

Note that "beating the clock" also doesn't mean that you shouldn't eat three square meals a day if that's what your body is telling you to do. If traditional meal times match your body's natural eating cycle, then by all means listen to your body. The goal here is to let your body, and not the clock, determine your eating cycle.

FOOD TRACKER

Complex carbohydrates and foods rich in protein tend to be more satisfying than other types of food.

Looking over the nutrition information in your Food Tracker, did you eat less when the food items were rich in protein or complex carbohydrates?

Which food items had the highest satisfaction score? For these items, what was their protein and complex carbohydrate score? How does their calorie content relate to the other numbers?

As you look back over your Food Tracker, can you tell when you ate each item? It may be helpful to add a column for time of day for each food item on the list, or just make an effort to notice when you're eating.

Are you more likely to be hungry in the morning, in the afternoon, or in the evening? Do you find yourself "midnight snacking?" If so, when were you eating throughout the day that day?

The more you become aware of which foods satisfy your hunger, and when, the more you will be able to practice conscious eating.

KEY POINTS TO REMEMBER FOR LESSON 6

- Eat when you are hungry; stop when you are satisfied

- Hunger is a physical sensation; appetite is a craving of the mind

- Conscious eating means paying attention to your body's natural hunger signals

- "Beat the Clock" by eating when you are hungry, and not because the clock says it's meal time

- Notice the nutritional content of the food you're eating, and which items have the highest satisfaction score

- Notice any patterns related to when you ate and whether or not you were satisfied by what you ate

REFERENCES

Cornell University: Big Meals vs. Mini Meals

https://www.concorde.edu/about-us/blog/health-care-insights/health-care-awareness-meal-size

LESSON 7

CALL A TRUCE

Calling a truce with the guilt induced by the diet mentality means giving yourself unconditional permission to eat. Unless there's a medical reason you shouldn't have certain foods, no food item is off the table.

This runs contrary to what we've been taught, and seems counter-intuitive, but if certain foods are off the table, that makes them increasingly irresistible.

What happens when we eliminate certain foods from our diet is that subconsciously our brains go into 'famine' mode. When your unconscious mind knows that food is available, then there's no rush to eat, because you can eat any time.

Imagine you're living in a hunter-gatherer society where food is not readily available 24 hours a day, 7 days a week. Abundant food is rare in such a situation. Our bodies and our brains evolved in just that type of environment.

If you're living in such a situation, the natural and logical thing to do is to binge whenever food is available, because you never know when you might have the opportunity to eat again, so your body eats as much as it can and stores up the energy in the form of fat. This reserve energy is available for use when food is not.

Now imagine, in the same type of society, you're living in a period where food is plentiful. There's no need to binge and store up food energy because you know the larder is full and you can eat any time you want. Since your unconscious mind knows this, it doesn't feel the need to prompt you to eat.

The diet mentality triggers your unconscious mind into famine mode. When you forbid certain foods, your brain and body naturally assume there's a famine. When you give in to a moment of weakness and make the food available, then your body's natural processes take over and your unconscious mind tells you to eat as much as possible, because your unconscious mind thinks that the food might never be available again.

The diet mentality puts your brain into a state of hyper focus. The unconscious mind is concerned with survival, and an element of survival is food.

In fact, food is one of the most basic, and therefore one of the most fundamental, components of survival. This hyper focus is compounded by the fact that your unconscious mind has no sense of time. It doesn't know that there might be food available tomorrow. It's only concerned with the fact that there's a delicious food readily available right here and right now, and it better take advantage of the fact, since there's no way of knowing if it will be available later. This is because your natural, unconscious survival processes have no concept of the future. They're only concerned with here and now.

The diet mentality leads to a never-ending cycle of restricting certain foods, then bingeing on them, then feeling guilty for bingeing. The feeling of guilt leads to restricting your diet even more, which triggers your unconscious survival instinct to eat even more food when bingeing, leading to even more guilt, and even more diet restrictions. So the cycle continues.

The way out of this cycle is to give yourself unconditional permission to eat.

If you allow yourself to eat whatever you want, whenever you want, won't that lead to out-of-control eating? My answer to that would be to ask if the diet mentality is giving you control over your eating. If you're stuck in the restrict-binge-guilt cycle, I'd say you're already out of control regarding your diet.

The definition of "insanity" is "doing the same things in the same way and expecting different results." If restricting your diet isn't working, then how would restricting it even more work?

Maybe it's time to try something different. You can do something different by calling a truce with your relationship to food.

Natural Eating

The key to natural eating is to give yourself permission to eat whatever your body naturally craves, while also paying attention to your body's natural satisfaction cues. This is accomplished in a five-step process.

Try this for the coming week and see what a difference it makes in calling a truce with the diet mentality.

STEP 1

Look at the food satisfaction score on your Food Tracker. That column indicates which foods give you the most satisfaction. You can use the "sort" function on your Food Glossary to rank the foods on your list from most satisfying to least satisfying, or simply make a mental note of which foods have the highest satisfaction scores.

STEP 2

Have you been restricting any of the foods on your Food Glossary list? What is their satisfaction score? Make a list of the foods with the highest satisfaction score that you eat most often. If you're restricting any foods on your Food Glossary, make a list of their satisfaction scores as well.

STEP 3

If you're restricting certain foods from your diet, then give yourself permission to eat them, and then go to the store and buy them. If you're not restricting any foods on your diet, congratulations! You're halfway to calling a truce with your food!

STEP 4

Use your mindful eating skills to allow yourself to savor the "forbidden" foods on your list. Focus on nothing but the sensations and experience of eating. Does the food still satisfy you as much as you imagined it would? Does savoring every bite in this manner while paying attention to your body's natural satisfaction cues help you to eat less of it? In short, are two bites of your favorite food more or less delicious than one bite?

STEP 5

Make sure you keep your pantry stocked with foods that are high on your satisfaction list. Even if you don't eat them frequently, it helps to quieten your unconscious mind's "famine" response just knowing they're readily available should you ever desire to eat them.

The key to natural eating is to learn your body's signals. If you learn to trust your body, it will tell you when it needs to be fed, and when it's time to stop eating.

When you learn to distinguish between hunger and appetite, you can call a truce with your food by only eating when you're hungry. When you learn to respond to your body's natural satisfaction cues, you can stop eating when you're satisfied.

This doesn't mean you have to limit or eliminate any foods from your pantry. It means you learn to eat naturally by respecting what your body is telling you.

FOOD TRACKER

Look again at your foods with the highest satisfaction scores. Now look at the nutrition information for each. How many are high in carbohydrates? In fats? In proteins? In calories?

Do you see any patterns and relationships between food satisfaction scores and nutritional information? What do these patterns tell you about which foods are satisfying to you?

Does your food satisfaction score for your favorite "forbidden" foods change when you complete the five steps outlined above?

POINTS TO REMEMBER FROM LESSON 7

- Give yourself unconditional permission to eat whatever you want whenever you want.

- Unless there's a medical reason to restrict your diet, all foods are literally "on the table."

- Restrictive dieting activates your body's "famine" response, leading to binge eating.

- Remember "quality and not quantity." Two bites of a food don't taste any better than one bite of food.

- Use your mindful skills to be aware of your body's natural satisfaction cues.

REFERENCES

Balance Health and Healing
Intuitive Eating 101: Make Peace with Food
https://balancehealthandhealing.com/intuitive-eating-101-make-peace-with-food/

LESSON 8

CHALLENGE THE FOOD POLICE

The Family Food Cop

If your family is like most, you have at least one "food cop." This person (or persons) has made it their duty to point out every time you eat something that they don't consider healthy. Although this person means well, what they don't realize is that their comments could be the very thing that triggers the guilt/binge cycle.

If you have such a person in your life, the first thing to do would be to show them some of the studies linked in this program so that they can see for themselves that their comments are having the opposite of the intention desired.

If that doesn't work, then the next thing to do is to set a firm but friendly boundary with them by saying something like, "I hear you, and I understand and appreciate your concern; however, I'm taking care of this on my own. While I appreciate your advice, I'd appreciate it if in the future you let me deal with it."

If you set a boundary with this person and they still persist on being your food cop, then it's time to recognize that their comments are more about their own control issues than about your behavior. Just thank them for their concern and move on.

Challenging the Food Police

Food cops don't just show up in families. They're also at work, in church, in social clubs, and even in your own head. Here are some common comments food cops make, and how to deal with them.

"You were so bad, you ate dessert."

Remember the only rule of losing weight is to burn more calories than you consume. If you allow yourself a dessert once in a while, there's absolutely nothing wrong with enjoying it. Just use your mindful skills to stop when you feel satisfied. Experiment with the idea of not forcing yourself to eat the whole dessert.

"Clean your plate!"

This is a common refrain among parents everywhere. The problem with hearing it often enough is that eventually we condition ourselves to keep eating long past the point we are satisfied. Natural eating means listening to your body's satisfaction cues and not feeling you have to eat all the food on your plate or finish your entire dessert. Trust your body to tell you when it's time to stop.

"I shouldn't eat anything past 6 p.m."

The only rule about when you should eat with natural eating is to eat when you are hungry. If you force your body's natural cycles into some arbitrary timetable of when you should and when you shouldn't eat, you may fall into the trap of forcing yourself to eat when you are not hungry. When that happens, the inevitable result is eating too much.

"Bread is bad for you."

Unless you have a medical reason to abstain from certain foods, there is no food that is "good" or "bad." If you have bread on occasion, just remember to use your mindful eating skills to get the most enjoyment possible out of it, and to be aware of your body's satisfaction signals.

"I won't lose weight if I eat that."

How much of it are you planning to eat? Are two bites of your favorite food more delicious than one bite if you savor every moment of the experience? Experiment with the idea that you don't have to eat the entire food item. You just have to eat until you're satisfied.

"I shouldn't eat fat...it's too high in calories."

Your body needs a certain amount of fat to survive. Once again, the rule of natural eating is that the only rule for weight loss is to consume fewer calories than you burn. If you burn fat calories after consuming them, you will lose weight.

The Food Police in Your Head

Living in a society permeated with the diet mentality, it's not surprising that we should internalize a lot of negative messages from the food police.

Try this...the next time you're eating, engage your mindful skills to observe and describe your self-talk regarding food.

Do you catch any negative self-talk? Are the food police in your head challenging you? If so, that's okay too. You can note the thought and let it go without having to act on it. Don't judge the thought as "good" or "Bad." It's simply a thought.

Remember that you are not your thoughts. Just because you are having a thought, that doesn't mean you have to act on it. It doesn't mean you have to believe the thought to be true.

The next time you hear a food cop's voice in your head, just note it without placing any judgment on it, and return to enjoying your food.

As you begin to become familiar with your internal dialog regarding the way you eat, notice how the beliefs you have about food and eating may influence your life.

Are there any "food cop" thoughts you're still clinging to? Do you find them hard to let go of? If so, why? Are the rules and beliefs your own internal food cop dispenses inside your head helping you to create a healthy, balanced life? Are they causing you to feel any guilt? Do you tend to binge eat when you feel guilty?

What thoughts and beliefs about food and eating might you wish to challenge? How could you replace those "food cop" thoughts with healthier alternatives? Do you have any irrational or unreasonable thoughts or beliefs about food? How could you change those to something more reasonable and rational?

As you challenge the food police, remember to use all six of your mindful skills to help you nurture yourself. Engage your compassionate side to be gentle with yourself and others as you go about making the changes you choose for your life.

The more you are able to do this, the more you'll create a new, more natural relationship with your food.

FOOD TRACKER

To practice challenging the food police, look at your food satisfaction scores on your Food Glossary.

Pick three of the foods with the highest satisfaction scores and give yourself permission to enjoy them sometime this coming week. Use your mindful skills to savor the experience and to stop when you are satisfied

POINTS TO REMEMBER FROM LESSON 8

- Deal with the "food cops" among your family and friends by setting healthy boundaries with them.

- Challenge the "food cop" in your own head by using your mindful skills.

- Just because you have a thought doesn't mean you have to believe it or act on it.

- The only rule for losing weight is to burn more calories than you consume.

- There are no "good" foods or "bad" foods.

- Give yourself permission to eat without judgment.

- Replace "food cop" thoughts with more rational and reasonable thoughts, using your mindful skills.

REFERENCES

Challenge the Food Police
https://www.evelyntribole.com/principle-4-challenge-the-food-police/

Well Made Nutrition
9 Ways to Challenge the Food Police
https://www.wellmadenutrition.com/blogposts/2019/9/23/10-ways-to-challenge-the-food-police

LESSON 9

CONNECT TO YOUR SENSES

Doing Mode and Being Mode

Mindfulness is a shift from Doing Mode to Being Mode. We often get trapped inside our own heads with "to do" lists that we worry about all day until everything is checked off. If you've ever caught your mind wandering, making it difficult to focus on a task, there's a good chance that your mind was trapped in Doing Mode.

By way of illustration, when you were in the shower this morning, were you really in the shower? Were you enjoying the pleasant sensations of the water on your skin, the smell of the soap, and the sounds of the running water? Or was your mind already five miles down the road at the office, thinking about what you have to do today?

If your answer was the latter, then your mind was stuck in Doing Mode.

Now imagine you're sitting down to enjoy a meal. Your mouth and hands are going through the motions of eating, but your mind is telling you to hurry up and eat because you have another project to do after the meal.

If you've ever had that experience, you can see how that could cause you not to enjoy your meal at all because you weren't actually there, present with the experience of enjoying your food. What's needed in such a situation is a shift from Doing Mode to Being Mode. In Being Mode, you can be present in the moment so that you can "be with" the pleasure of eating.

One way to shift from Doing Mode to Being Mode is to focus on the experiences your senses are giving you. It's a shift from Thinking Mode into Sensing Mode.

When you are able to leave those "to do" lists behind and to stop thinking about the future, you are able to pay more attention to what your senses are telling you. The reason focusing on your senses allows you to enter into Being Mode is that it's impossible to experience anything with your senses in the past or in the future. You can't taste something in the present that you ate a week ago. You can't smell something in the present that you will eat a week from now. You can't enjoy a past or future meal with your senses.

While you might be able to remember a pleasant meal and to look forward to eating it again, you can only experience a meal through your senses in the present moment. That's why focusing on your senses automatically brings you into Being Mode.

If your mind is wandering while you're eating, your focus is not on what your senses are telling you about the meal. If you're thinking about the next project, your mind is on the work involved in accomplishing that task, and not on the in-the-moment satisfaction of enjoying what you're eating.

Likewise, if you're eating while working on the computer, or while watching television, or reading, your mind is on that and not on enjoying the meal.

The way out of this "mind trap" is to learn to eat with all five of your senses.

Eating with Your Senses

My undergraduate degree was in Experimental Psychology. One of the experiments we conducted in the lab was how visual cues are related to your experience of food. We asked participants what their favorite foods were, then prepared the dishes for them, but with one critical difference: The appearance of the food was altered in some way. For example, one participant loved mashed potatoes.

We prepared mashed potatoes for her according to her favorite recipe, but with one critical difference. We used food coloring to turn them blue. Upon seeing the blue mashed potatoes she couldn't eat them because they "tasted funny."

Just to make sure that there wasn't something in the food coloring that was altering the tastes of the potatoes, we had her sample two dishes while blindfolded. One dish contained the potatoes with the blue food coloring, and the other was from the same batch without the food coloring. While blindfolded, she couldn't tell the difference and said that they both tasted fine.

The conclusion was that just by altering the color of the mashed potatoes, her experience of eating them was altered. This is just one way that our senses can impact our satisfaction with food.

Because we live in a fast-paced society, we've convinced ourselves that we don't have time to actually sit down and enjoy a meal. Taking the time to experience a meal in Being Mode with all your senses can be difficult, but it's not impossible. The benefits are well worth the effort, and with a little practice it's not really as time-consuming as it may seem.

Until you get a little practice with eating with your senses, you may want to set aside a special time to try this for the first time. Choose a time and a place where you will be undisturbed for the duration of the meal. This should be at least thirty minutes, depending on the size of the meal you're enjoying, but there are no hard and fast rules as long as you're able to focus on your senses for the length of the meal, no matter how long it takes.

Pause for a moment and think about how you experience food with all of your senses. Then, when you're ready to try this experiment, sit down with your meal, eliminate all distractions, and then explore the experience of eating using the guidelines below for each sense.

SIGHT

Put down your fork or spoon and take the time to look closely at the meal. Notice the colors, the shapes, and the textures. What about the arrangement of the food on the plate makes it appealing to you?

Based solely on what you're seeing, which food item would you like to try first? How does what you're seeing enhance your satisfaction with the meal?

SMELL

Close your eyes and take a deep breath. What pleasant aromas do you notice first? Could you identify this meal simply through your sense of smell? Can you distinguish between multiple food items on your plate using only your sense of smell? Do the aromas you're sensing evoke any pleasant memories or associations?

TOUCH

Lift the plate or bowl and hold it in your hands. Do you sense any difference in temperature after picking it up? How heavy is the container with the food in it?

If there are food items on the plate that you can eat with your fingers, pick one up and feel the texture. Is it smooth or rough? Does it have any ridges or protrusions? Could you identify this item solely using your sense of touch?

If you need to use a fork or a spoon, pick up a bite and notice if it's heavy or light. What's the smallest amount you could feel on your fork or spoon that you would still be able to taste if you put it in your mouth?

TASTE

Bring a bite of food up to your lips, but don't put it into your mouth yet. Are you starting to salivate in anticipation? Now place the item on your tongue.

There are four types of taste bud; sweet, sour, salt and bitter. As you begin to slowly chew the food, which of these tastes do you notice first? Where on your tongue do you first taste the food?

As you chew slowly, does the texture of the food change? Continue to chew and enjoy the flavors of the food.

When you're ready, swallow. Before you take another bite, pause for a moment to allow your taste buds to clear before taking another bite. It may help to put down your fork or spoon for a moment.

HEARING

If you're eating a crunchy food, listen to the sounds it makes as you chew it. What do the sounds add to the enjoyment of your meal?

If it's a softer texture of food, listen for any subtle sounds your body might be making as you eat it. If it's soup, do you slurp it? If it's pudding or mashed potatoes or something of a similar texture, do your lips smack together as you chew?

Does your throat make any noise as you swallow? How about your stomach?

After the Meal

When you connect with your senses like this while enjoying a meal, you may notice that you eat less because you enjoy your food more, and you can be satisfied with less.

Don't fall into the trap of thinking that you must finish it all just because it's on your plate. Stop when you are satisfied.

One way to experiment with this idea is to automatically divide your food in half while it's on your plate. When you eat the first half, ask yourself if you really need to eat the second half, or are you satisfied?

When you are done eating, pause for a moment to savor the meal. It may help to close your eyes and rest your hands on your thighs. Put your fork or spoon down, take a couple of deep breaths and center yourself.

What was the most enjoyable portion of the meal? What was the least enjoyable? Did you have any emotional sensations during the meal? What were they? Why do you think that the meal evoked those emotions?

Did you have any memories regarding this meal? What were they? Why do you think the meal recalled these memories?

Did experiencing your food with all of your senses change your satisfaction with the meal? If so, how?

Sensory Integration Meditation

For more practice with integrating your senses into not only eating, but all aspects of your life, try the Sensory Integration Meditation outlined below.

Before beginning the meditation, first make sure you are in a place where you will be undisturbed for the duration of the meditation.

Next, find a comfortable position, either sitting or lying down. If you are wearing any tight or restrictive clothing, you may wish to loosen it or change into something more comfortable.

When you are ready to begin, read over the instructions below, then try do meditation. If you have a way of recording yourself you may wish to make a recording to listen to as you participate in the activity.

This meditation is especially effective if you practice it at the table prior to engaging in a meal. If you're not eating alone you can invite your friends or family members to join you. Afterwards you can discuss how the meditation might have changed your experience of the meal.

- Start by closing your eyes and taking a few deep cleansing breaths.

- As you feel the air entering your lungs, you are breathing in calmness and relaxation.

- As you exhale, allow worries, tension and stress to evaporate from your body, mind and spirit.

- Allow yourself to enter into a state of mindful awareness for a time, focusing only on your breathing.

- Remember that if at any time during this Sensory Integration Meditation you should encounter thoughts or feelings that are overwhelming to you, you should stop the meditation and return to it when you are calmer.

- When you are ready, allow your attention to focus around the sensation of the air flowing into your nostrils as you inhale. Feel the air entering your nasal passages.

- As you direct your attention to your nose, do you notice any aromas? Are they pleasant odors or pungent odors? Do the scents you find around you evoke any memories?

- If you are doing this meditation prior to enjoying a meal, focus on the aromas of the food you're about to eat. Close your eyes and focus only on the scents. Could you identify the meal solely by its aroma?

- If you encounter a fragrance that triggers a happy memory, allow that happiness to embrace and envelope you.

- Linger here for a while with the aromas you find around you.

- When you are ready to move on, direct your attention to your mouth and tongue. As your breath leaves your body with each exhalation, do you detect any taste on your breath? It may be a subtle sensation, or not noticeable at all.

- If it is not a noticeable sensation, that's okay too. If it is noticeable, describe what sort of taste it is. Is it sweet or bitter? Sour or salty? How does it compare to the fragrances you smell right now?

- Try to 'smell' the food using your tongue. Does this change the experience in any way?

- Move your attention now to your ears. What do you hear? Are there any background noises? If you're eating with others, can you hear them moving around you? If eating alone, what sounds do you notice in the nearby environment?

- Can you hear the sound of your breathing?

- Can you hear the sound of your own heart beating?

- Focus for a moment on the information your ears bring to you.

- Move your attention now to your body. If you are sitting at the table when doing this meditation, notice how your body makes contact with the chair.

- Pay attention to all of the sensations you're experiencing in your body right now. Can you detect any physiological changes in anticipation of eating? Is your mouth watering? Is your stomach rumbling?

- Are there any pressure points of contact between your body and the chair? Or the table?

- Do you feel pressure from any tight clothing?

- Overall, are you comfortable, or is there some tension somewhere in your body?

- Can you melt the tension away by focusing your attention on it?

- Can you tell whether you're experiencing hunger or appetite?

- Now move your attention to your eyes. If they are still closed, open them slowly, giving them time to adjust to the light.

- As you observe your meal, see the food without assumptions, in a new way.

- Imagine yourself an artist. If you were to paint or draw the meal you see before you, how would you capture the detail you see?

- Observe the variations in color, shading and light that you see in the food. Focus on the spaces between the food items rather than on the foods themselves.

- If you were asked to draw only the spaces you see before you, what would that look like?

- Examine every detail of everything you see before you.

- Now close your eyes again and come back to yourself.

- Gradually allow your attention and consciousness to expand to your surroundings.

- Did this meditation evoke any memories, thoughts or feelings? If so, note them for consideration after this meditation is over.

- As you bring your awareness back to yourself, note how you are feeling right now. Remember this feeling when the meditation is done.

- Return your attention only to your breathing. Feel the air enter and leave your body.

- When you feel you are ready, open your eyes again and end the meditation feeling calm yet invigorated.

- If you are at the table, go ahead and eat, carrying this mindful awareness with you by focusing on one thing at a time. Enjoy each bite of your food as it comes to you.

FOOD TRACKER

Try the meditation above at least once in the coming week. Now pick 2 or 3 of your favorite foods from your food tracker, based on their satisfaction scores.

If you choose to eat any of those items in the coming week, try the Sensory Integration Meditation prior to eating them, and then use the guidelines from the Eating with Your Senses section above.

Did your experience of the food change?

KEY POINTS TO REMEMBER FOR LESSON 9

- Mindfulness is a shift from Doing Mode to Being Mode

- One way to shift from Doing Mode to Being Mode is to shift from Thinking Mode to Sensing Mode

- In Being Mode, you can be with the pleasure of enjoying a meal without any distractions

- You can only experience a meal through your senses in the present moment

- To escape the "mind trap" of Doing Mode, learn to eat with all five of your senses

- When you connect with your senses while enjoying a meal, you may notice that you eat less because you enjoy your food more, and you can be satisfied with less

REFERENCES

Altamore, Luca & Ingrassia, Marzia & Chironi, Stefania & Columba, Pietro & Sortino, Giuseppe & Vukadin, Ana & Bacarella, Simona. (2018). Pasta experience: Eating with the five senses-A pilot study. *AIMS*

Agriculture and Food. 3. 493-520. 10.3934/agrfood.2018.4.493.

LESSON 10

COMFORT YOUR FEELINGS, NOT YOUR APPETITE

My grandparents were farmers who lived through the Great Depression. Surviving this experience meant they knew what it was like to be truly hungry.

When the Depression ended, having food on the table meant success to them. Whenever I visited them, the first question they always asked was, "Are you hungry?" One of the ways they demonstrated love was by meeting one of the most basic needs of life. Every family gathering featured a feast.

There were even special foods for special occasions. I remember my grandmother buying a single pomegranate every holiday season. This pomegranate was shared with everyone at the table. To her, it symbolized wealth and success, and the desire to give the best to her family and friends.

Think about all the good times you've had with friends and family. How many of those experiences involved food in some way? Even if it didn't feature a full meal, were there snacks available at the event? What were your family's messages concerning food?

Our most basic needs are food, clothing, shelter, and love. Food is a basic and fundamental need. That's why people with process addictions to food can't quit "cold turkey." We have to eat to live.

One of the most fundamental ways our parents can express their love to us is by feeding us. Sometimes this turns into "more love means more food" Because of this it's only logical that our thoughts, feelings, and beliefs around food should involve an element of emotional comfort.

If you're like most people, gatherings with family and friends feature food in some way. Food means love. Food means companionship. Food means fellowship. Food means comfort.

Comfort Foods

The next time you have a craving for a certain food and you're not hungry, ask yourself why. Stop for a moment and ask yourself, "What am I feeling right now?"

Be totally honest about your current emotional state. Use your mindful skills to shift from Doing Mode into Being Mode.

Remember, eating is "doing." In Being Mode you can just sit and be with the craving until it subsides.

Next, engage your mindful skills of observing, describing, and participating to allow yourself to experience the emotional sensations that come with the craving.

If you have an appetite for a particular food, ask yourself what emotional associations that particular food has for you. Can you remember the first time you ate it, and what feelings that experience generated in you? Was it a sensation of comfort? Are you craving this food because you need comforting right now? Is there another way you could find such comfort?

Auto-Pilot

Driving a car on the open road for the first time can be an overwhelming experience. There's a lot of information you're responsible for. You have to remember which pedals do what. You have to remember what all the signs mean. You have to remember what all the lines on the road mean. You have to watch for other drivers, for pedestrians, and for other potential road hazards like potholes and rain or sleet on the road.

If you're like most people you were probably very nervous the first time you had to drive by yourself.

But over time, and with practice, you soon learned to master the vehicle. In fact, experienced drivers often go into "auto-pilot" mode and don't have to actually think very much about the process of driving.

If you've ever had the experience of driving past your exit because you were on auto-pilot, you're familiar with this idea.

The challenge with comforting your feelings and not your appetite is that often our emotional processes go on auto-pilot as well. The first time you have an emotional reaction to something, you have a belief about the experience, then you act on that belief, then you get a consequence.

For example, the first time someone does something that hurts your feelings, it's perfectly natural to seek comfort. If no other avenues of comfort-seeking are available, you might look around for something to eat.

Given the reasons outlined above that food is linked with comfort, food is often the "go to" resource for quick, but temporary, comfort. So you might have a belief like, "If I eat something, I'll feel better."

So you eat a comfort food, and then you feel better. At least for a while. But too much comfort eating results in the consequence of being overweight or unhealthy. Not only that, but it doesn't deal with the real emotional need that led you to seek a comfort food in the first place.

This difficulty is compounded by the fact that if you follow this pattern long enough, the process tends to become automatic, like driving a car. When the process of dealing with emotions goes into auto-pilot mode, it's easy to gloss over the belief that led to the action.

When this happens, the belief has become an unconscious process. So for example, if the belief is, "If I eat something I'll feel better," then over time that belief goes into auto-pilot and you don't even think about it before reaching for a comfort food.

Once it has become an unconscious, auto-pilot response, it'll take a little practice to become consciously aware of the belief that led to the craving in the first place.

Don't get discouraged if you have to practice this for a while before succeeding. If it were easy you'd already be doing it!

Remember to cease the diet mentality while examining the need for comfort foods using your mindful skills. If you can do this, then over time you can cease going into auto-pilot mode when it comes to food.

Comfort Your Feelings

Assuming that your craving for comfort in food is based on appetite, and not hunger, the next step is to ask yourself what other comforts might suffice to meet your emotional needs other than resorting to food. What is your body really telling you that it wants? What emotion needs comforting?

This is where the "how" skills of mindfulness can be a big help.

First ask yourself if you are making any judgments or assumptions about the situation. An example of an assumption might be, "I need comforting, and food is the only answer."

This is one of those auto-pilot beliefs that might need closer examination. Practice your mindful skill of being non-judgmental to look at the assumptions and beliefs you've made about the situation. Are there any assumptions that need challenging?

Now use your mindful skill of focusing on one thing at a time (being one-mindful) to consider the craving. Do you really need this food right now, or is it just a want? If you can sit with the craving until it subsides, can you find another way to meet your emotional needs? What might that way be?

Finally, focus your mindful power of intention to effectively find an alternative resolution. Remember, the two questions of intent are:

1. What is my intention in this situation?

2. Is what I'm about to do going to support that intention?

If your intention is to practice natural eating by only eating when you are hungry, is giving in to a craving or an appetite going to accomplish that intention?

When you're able to use all your mindful skills in this manner, you will have learned to comfort your feelings instead of your appetite.

FOOD TRACKER

How many "comfort foods" can you find on your Food Tracker?

How does their satisfaction score compare with other foods on your list?

Does this information help you to comfort your feelings instead of your appetite?

POINTS TO REMEMBER FROM LESSON 10

- In most families and at most social events, food means love and comfort

- Appetite and cravings are usually the result of an emotional need that needs comforting

- The next time you have a craving, stop and ask yourself, "What am I feeling right now?"

- Our emotional processes often go on auto-pilot; this is when we seek comfort foods

- If you feel yourself going into auto-pilot mode, use your mindful skills to explore the feeling and the craving, then shift into Being Mode until it subsides

- Ask yourself what other ways there might be to seek emotional comfort

REFERENCES

Christiana Institute of Advanced Surgery
Emotional Eating & How to Stop It
http://www.umusa.net/wellnessprograms/medicalweightloss/handouts/E
    motional%20Eating.pdf

LESSON 11

CHOOSE CHANGE

Forming New Habits

According to a 2009 study on how habits are formed, on average it takes 66 days for a new behavior to become a habit. Depending on the type of habit, the range is from 18 days to 254 days.

This wide range can be narrowed down depending on the type of habit you're trying to develop. According to the National Institute of Health, the hardest habits to change are those related to pleasure. This is because pleasure-related habits produce dopamine in the brain.

Dopamine is the brain's "happy juice." The more dopamine a habit produces in your brain, the more you feel rewarded for engaging in that habit and the more you crave the dopamine "fix" of doing it again.

You may recall at the beginning of the Natural Eating program that change happens when one of two things happens:

1. Either the pain of staying the same becomes greater than the pain of changing; or,

2. The pleasure of changing becomes greater than the pleasure of staying the same.

How does this relate to the process of replacing old habits with new ones? You can't form a new habit until the pleasure of the new habit becomes greater than the pleasure of the old habit.

This means that if you want to permanently change your relationship with food, you have to find a way to increase the amount of pleasure you get from Natural Eating or decrease the amount of pleasure you got from your former way of eating.

According to the aforementioned 2009 study, the way to reduce the number of days that it takes to form a new habit is to increase the number of repetitions of the new habit and decrease the number of repetitions of the old habit until the old habit is completely eliminated.

Since eating is a pretty regular habit, you have at least three opportunities per day to practice the tools and techniques of Natural Eating. The study concluded that on average it takes 66 days to form a new habit. If you have been following the Natural Eating program and completing the exercises every week, then at this point in the program you have had 70 days to practice. By the end of the program you will have had 84 days to practice.

This means that if you've made it this far, the chances of making permanent change are in your favor.

If you still have an occasional relapse into old behaviors, like occasional binge-eating or eating past the point of satisfaction, that's okay too.

Research shows that people relapse an average of three times before making lasting, permanent change.

Give yourself permission to learn and grow, just as you've learned to give yourself permission to eat. Congratulations on making it this far! You're almost there!

Types of Habits

There are four main types of habits. If you're working on replacing old habits with new ones, it helps to review the types and to be familiar with which types you're replacing.

Let's review the types, what they are, and how to change them using the techniques of Natural Eating

1) Habits of Desire

A habit of desire is a pattern of behavior that starts with a craving for something, and ends with a reward. It could be a desire for food, or alcohol, or drugs, or sexual gratification, or any other activity that stimulates your brain's dopamine response.

The way to change such a habit is to replace the dopamine reward of the old habit with a habit that has a dopamine reward of an equal or higher value.

In Natural Eating, the habit can manifest as a desire to eat too much of a favorite food. Notice that in Natural Eating, it's not the desire of the food itself that is the problem, since no foods are off the table unless there's a medical reason for not eating it.

The problem with the habit comes in when we eat past the point of satisfaction. If you were actually able to see what was going on in the dopamine-producing section of your brain while eating a favorite food, you'd see that past a certain point your brain reaches a point of diminishing returns.

What that means is that when you bite into your favorite food item, your brain produces a rush of dopamine, but as you continue to eat more and more of it, the dopamine-producing centers of your brain produce less and less dopamine, until your brain is no longer rewarding you for indulging.

If you give yourself permission to eat your favorite foods, and then to stop when you've reached the point of satisfaction, then you've trained your brain and your body to stop eating when the dopamine production has peaked and has started to diminish.

The easiest way to stop when you're satisfied is to connect with your senses while eating (see Lesson 10) and eat one bite at a time. After each bite, ask yourself, "Am I satisfied yet?" If the answer is "now," then you can continue eating, but if the answer is "yes," then it's time to stop.

2) Habits of Distraction

A habit of distraction is a habit you tend to automatically fall into without thinking about it, as a distraction while you're engaged in another behavior.

In Natural Eating, unconscious eating is a habit of distraction.

Suppose you keep a jar of candy on your desk and you keep absentmindedly reaching for it while working. If you've ever done this, you've engaged in a habit of distraction.

The way to change a habit of distraction is to practice Conscious Eating as described in Lesson 6. Replace automatic, unconscious thought processes about food and eating with conscious, intentional and intuitive eating habits.

3) Habits of Emotion

A habit of emotion is similar to a habit of distraction in that it is a tendency to engage in certain habitual behaviors in response to emotions.

The difference is that we engage in a habit of distraction when we're occupied with something else, but we engage in a habit of emotion to avoid having to experience the emotion directly. In my house we used to call it "eating at somebody."

Suppose I got angry at my wife for some reason, and instead of dealing with the anger, I instead went in the fridge and at a half-gallon of ice cream. At those times, my rationale was, "Well, she made me mad, so I deserve to eat this!"

In my mind, I had relieved myself of the responsibility for dealing with my own emotional eating by shifting the blame onto my wife. If you've ever done anything similar, instead of asking, "what's eating me?" instead ask yourself, "Who am I eating at?"

Sometimes it's not a person that we're eating at. Sometimes it may be a situation, or just an overall mood. In those times, ask yourself if you really want food, or if you're just yielding to a habit of emotion. Then deal with the emotion in other ways instead of reaching for food.

One way to do this is to ask yourself, "What am I experiencing right now?" and to be honest with yourself about the answer. Remember to use your mindful skills and to not place any judgments on whatever answers you find. You feel what you feel. There's no such thing as a "wrong" or a "bad" feeling.

What matters is how you choose to respond to the feeling. You can just allow yourself to experience the feeling in Being Mode without having to "do" anything about it. That includes not reaching for comfort foods when your emotions are in play.

4) Habits of Doing

The fourth and final type of habit is a habit of doing. Habits of doing are not always bad things. If you've made it this far in the Natural Eating program, you're working towards building new, healthier relationships with food, so in this case a habit of doing is a good thing. there are, however, some types of habits that are habits of doing.

When I was a smoker, I had a habit of having a cigarette with my morning coffee and a cigarette after every meal. Most of the time it wasn't even that I wanted a cigarette. It was just a habit that formed over time.

Another habit of doing might be always having a dessert after dinner, or eating everything on your plate even though you stopped being hungry halfway through the meal, or eating a whole candy bar just because you unwrapped it.

When we have certain thoughts and beliefs, and then we act on them, we get a result. If that result increases our pleasure or enjoyment or decreases our pain or discomfort, then we tend to repeat that behavior.

Do it often enough and it becomes a habit of doing. At some point, the process becomes automatic and we don't even think about it when indulging it, just like when I automatically lit a cigarette with my morning coffee.

The way to break a habit of doing is to become consciously aware of the thought processes that led us to indulge in it. If you suddenly find yourself nibbling on snacks, re-trace your steps until you can remember what triggered the behavior, then deal with the trigger using your mindful skills.

It takes time to form a habit of doing, so don't be discouraged if you can't break it after the first attempt. Commit to continue practicing your Natural Eating skills and eventually you'll replace your habit of doing with a more productive and healthier habit.

You may notice as you go over this list of habits that there's a lot of overlap. Don't get caught up in trying to figure out which type of habit is at play.

What's more important is focusing on how to deal with the problems they generate as they arise. As a general rule, when we reach for something to eat out of habit or in response to an emotion, it's because we seek the temporary relief and enjoyment that the food can bring. But an even longer-lasting enjoyment that is more permanent and healthy is to deal with the trigger that led us to reach for the food in the first place.

With each of these habits, the way to begin to deal with breaking the cycle is to shift from Doing Mode to Being Mode. In the present moment we can greet the impulse with an open and accepting attitude, without judgment. When this becomes a habit, you'll have mastered the skills of Natural Eating.

Statement of Purpose and Change Plan

In Lesson 2 you completed a *Statement of Purpose* and a *Change Plan*. The Statement of Purpose outlined why you want to change your relationship with food, and the Change Plan outlined how you planned to do it. The

Statement of Purpose is the "what" you want to do, and the Change Plan is "how" you want to do it.

If you have those handy, go over the questions below and see what you've learned so far in the Natural Eating program. You may wish to keep them nearby in the coming weeks and months as you replace your old habits with new Natural Eating habits.

Statement of Purpose

Get out your Statement of Purpose and answer the following questions.

- What reasons did you list on your Statement of Purpose for wanting to change your relationship with food?

- Have any of those reasons changed? How?

- Do you need to complete a new Statement of Purpose to reflect those changes?

- Review the Stages of Change from Lesson 2. For the items listed on your Statement of Purpose, have any of the Stages of Change shifted since you completed your Statement of Purpose?

- If so, how and why?

- Look at the *Motivations for Change* section on your Statement of Purpose. Look at the column marked, *Increasing the Pain of Staying the Same*. Would you answer differently now that you have completed most of the program?

- Do the same for the column marked, *Increasing the Pleasure of Changing*. Would any of those answers change now that you have a better understanding of Natural Eating?

Change Plan

Now let's look at your Change Plan. Review your answers on your Change Plan and answer the following questions.

- Are you making progress on the changes you wanted to make?

- Has your plan for making these changes been modified over the course of the Natural Eating program?

- If so, how?

- Were these changes an improvement?

- Where it says, "I will know my plan is working when this happens," you were asked to list some changes that would indicate that your change plan is working. Have any of those changes occurred?

- If so, what would you need to do make those changes permanent?

- If not, what would need to change in the way you're implementing the Natural Eating program to make those changes happen?

- Have you encountered anything that interfered with your ability to make your desired changes?

- If so, did your plan for dealing with those things work to your satisfaction?

- If not, what would have to be modified on your Change Plan to make that happen?

- There were three scaling questions at the bottom of the Change Plan. They're repeated below. Ask yourself these questions again, and rate yourself again on each, using the scale provided on the Change Plan.

- Did your numbers change?

- If so, did you see any improvement?

How to Make a Permanent Change

If you don't know that a problem exists, then you can't change it. The first step to making permanent and lasting change is to become aware of the problem.

The next step is to do something about it.

The final step is to make that change a habit. Zindel Segal, co-founder of the Mindfulness-Based Cognitive Therapy (MBCT) program, has identified seven drivers of old habits of thinking. These are:

1. Living on "automatic pilot" (rather than with awareness and conscious choice).

2. Relating to experience through thought (rather than directly sensing).

3. Dwelling on and in the past and future (rather than being fully in the present moment).

4. Trying to avoid, escape, or get rid of unpleasant experience (rather than approach it with interest).

5. Needing things to be different from how they are (rather than allowing them to be just as they already are).

6. Seeing thoughts as true and real (rather than as mental events that may or may not correspond to reality).

7. Treating yourself harshly and unkindly (rather than taking care of yourself with kindness and compassion).

Think about the habit(s) you want to change. Now become consciously aware of the habit by reading the list above.

What situations or events trigger the habit? Are there any thoughts or behaviors you could engage in that would help you to avoid indulging in the habit? When you feel the desire to engage in the habit, pay attention to what was going on at the time you experienced the trigger. Where were you? What were you doing? What were you feeling? What were you thinking? How is your body feeling? Are you experiencing any stressful sensations like a tightening of the chest or shallow and rapid breathing? Do you feel any tension anywhere in your body?

Take a few deep breaths and turn your attention inward to your emotional state. When have you felt like this before? What did you do when you felt that way? Are there any times when you felt this way but you avoided the temptation to indulge in your coping mechanism of comfort eating? Would what you did then help you to avoid the temptation again now?

Boredom is usually a sign that you've gotten stuck in auto-pilot. These auto-pilots times are danger zones for slipping into old habits. Whenever you feel bored, try something new. Go for a walk. Take up a new hobby. Read a book. Play a sport. Experiment with things that will satisfy you more than falling back into eating for comfort.

You might also take up the practice of daily meditation. There are several meditation recording in the Resources section of the Mindfulness-Based Ecotherapy website at www.mindfulecotherapy.org, or you can search online for guided mindful meditations.

If you've never meditated before, it may feel weird or strange to you at first, and that's okay too. If it didn't feel strange, you'd already be doing it.

Try doing a brief meditation for a few minutes each day for a month or two and see if it helps you to meet your goals. Studies have shown that regular meditation strengthens and re-wires your brain in the areas responsible for attention, concentration, impulse control, and making good decisions, so incorporating a daily meditation practice into your routine can help greatly when it comes to making changes in your lifestyle.

Try it at least once a day and see if it helps you to achieve your goals!

FOOD TRACKER

This is the 11th week of the Natural Eating program. If you have been completing your Food Tracker on a regular basis, you should have enough data now to notice patterns and trends.

Has your experience of food changed over the course of the program? How had your overall calorie intake changed since you began the program 11 weeks ago? Have your fat and protein intakes changed any? What about your carbohydrate and sugar intakes? Can you spot any pattern regarding these changes as they relate to your overall food satisfaction scores? Has your relationship with food changed over the course of the program? Have you learned to be more satisfied with less food?

POINTS TO REMEMBER FROM LESSON 11

- Repetition is the key to forming new habits. The more often you engage in a behavior, the sooner it will become a habit.

- There's no such thing as a "wrong" or a "bad" feeling. What matters is how you choose to respond to the feeling.

- After each bite, ask yourself, "Am I satisfied yet?" If the answer is "now," then you can continue eating, but if the answer is "yes," then it's time to stop.

- Replace automatic, unconscious thought processes about food and eating with conscious, intentional and intuitive eating habits.

- The next time you feel the desire to engage in emotional eating, instead of asking, "what's eating me?" instead ask yourself, "Who am I eating at?"

- When we have certain thoughts and beliefs, and then we act on them, we get a result. If that result increases our pleasure or enjoyment or decreases our pain or discomfort, then we tend to repeat that behavior. Do it often enough and it becomes a habit of doing.

- The first step to making permanent and lasting change is to become aware of the problem. The next step is to do something about it. The final step is to make that change a habit.

REFERENCES

Journal of the American Heart Association
Moderate-to-Vigorous Physical Activity and All-Cause Mortality: Do Bouts Matter?
https://www.ahajournals.org/doi/10.1161/JAHA.117.007678

These results provide evidence that mortality risk reductions associated with moderate to vigorous physical activity are independent of how activity is accumulated and can impact the development of physical activity guidelines and inform clinical practice.

Lally, P., Van Jaarsveld, C.H.M., Potts, H.W.W., Wardle, J. (2009). How are habits formed: Modelling habit formation in the real world, *European Journal of Social Psychology*.

National Institutes of Health
Breaking Bad Habits: Why It's So Hard to Change
https://newsinhealth.nih.gov/2012/01/breaking-bad-habits

Seven Drivers of Old Habits of Thinking
https://www.mindful.org/the-7-drivers-of-old-habits-of-thinking/

LESSON 12

MAINTAINING

If you've completed all 11 of the previous lessons, you now have all the skills you need to change your relationship with food using Natural Eating. If you've been using the skills, you should have already seen some results. Now, as we near the end of our journey, all that remains is to consistently implement those skills so that you get consistent results.

In Lesson 2 we discussed the Stages of Change. The final stage is...

> *Maintenance* - Once you've engaged in troubleshooting, fixed all the potential bugs in your solution, and found a plan that works, you're in the maintenance phase. This means that you're able to continue implementing your change plan successfully by increasing the pain of staying the same while increasing the pleasure of changing.

In this final lesson of the Natural Eating program, we'll talk about some potential problems that could come up as you continue Natural Eating, and how to deal with them.

When you're able to apply these troubleshooting skills consistently, you will have achieved the *Maintenance* phase of the Stages of Change.

Suppose I tell myself, "Changing my relationship with food is too hard. I can't do it!"

Does having that thought make it a fact?

The lesson here is that we are not our thoughts. We are not our feelings. We are something else. What this means is that just because we're having thoughts, that doesn't mean we have to listen to them.

It doesn't mean we have to believe them. Thoughts are just thoughts. You don't have to listen to your mind or let it push you around. The choice is always up to you.

When we make assumptions, those assumptions change our perceptions. When we change our perceptions, we change our reality. If I assume, "changing my relationship with food is too hard," then that alters my perception filter to only look for evidence that affirms my assumption that "change is too hard."

Over time, that means that eventually I will ignore any evidence to the contrary, so that I only see the evidence that confirms my assumption that change is too hard. When I can't see any evidence to the contrary, I create a reality for myself in which change is too hard, and I give up.

Now suppose I assume that "Yes, change is hard, but I've already made some changes so I know that it is possible to change."

What would that do to my perceptions? Would it help me to look for evidence that change can happen? Over time, what would that do to create a different reality in my life?

If you "slip up" from time to time and succumb to the temptation to binge eat, remember your mindful skill of being non-judgmental. Occasional binge eating doesn't mean you're a "bad" person or a "failure." It just means you're a human being who's learning and growing. As you give yourself permission to eat, also give yourself permission to be a human being.

Pick yourself up, dust yourself off, and get back on that horse. One binge-eating day isn't an excuse to give up. Change happens over time. What we're looking for here is long-term change. One day of binge-eating is not going to have a significant impact on weeks or months of natural eating.

Up until you started the Natural Eating program, you'd spent your whole life developing your relationship with food. It is only in the past 12 weeks that you have begun to change that relationship. Nobody is saying that it will be easy, but if you believe it will be impossible, then it will be. On the other hand, if you believe you can do it, you will succeed.

Exercise

You may have noticed that we haven't mentioned exercise much in this program up until now. There's a reason for that.

According to a systematic review of studies by Carla E. Cox (2017), subjects who used exercise alone for weight reduction experienced minimal weight loss. Many gained the weight back over time, with some even weighing more than they had when they started the exercise program.

Why is this?

Remember the only rule of losing weight is to burn more calories than you take in. While people like to think that exercise burns calories, people routinely overestimate the amount of calories it burns.

For example, the average candy bar contains 240 calories, as does the average 20-ounce soda. To burn off 240 calories, you'd have to do one of the following:

- Walk 10,000 steps (approximately five miles)

- Do 300 pushups

- Do an hour of jumping jacks

- Ride a bicycle at 15 mph for 30 minutes

- Swim fast for 30 minutes

- 30-45 minutes of aerobic exercise

- 40 minutes of intensive yard work

As you can see, if you rely solely on exercise as a weight loss strategy, without modifying your relationship with food in any way, you're going to be doing a lot of exercise!

Also, when exercise is your only method of weight loss, what happens if it's raining? Or if you get sick? Or if you have to work late? Or if anything else interferes with your schedule, causing you to miss a workout? Does that mean you just don't get to eat that day?

Of course this doesn't mean that you shouldn't exercise. Exercise is an important part of a healthy lifestyle. The lesson here is just don't rely on it as your sole means of controlling your weight. Exercise because it's good for you, and not because you want to lose weight.

Two major barriers to establishing a healthy workout routine are getting started and staying motivated. Over the years I've found that there are mindful ways around these problems.

To address the first problem, getting started, I use the two-minute rule. There's an old saying that a journey of a thousand miles begins with a single step. If you think about the thousand miles, you'll psych yourself out and you'll never even take the first step.

But if you just tell yourself you'll take the first step then see how you feel after that, you can take the next step, and the next, until you've done as many steps as you can for the day. Using this method, you've eventually completed a thousand-mile journey.

If I set a goal of working out for an hour every day at the gym, the hardest part is actually getting to the gym. I start thinking about how long an hour is, and how much effort I'll have to put in, so I never even get started. I find an excuse not to go.

That's where the two-minute rule comes in. What I do is tell myself, "I only have to do it for two minutes. If I don't feel like continuing after that, I can stop at any time." This gets me over the hardest part of the workout: Actually getting started!

I usually find that once I've done my two minutes of exercise, I just tell myself, "two more minutes," and keep doing that until I'm done, always giving myself permission to stop after "two more minutes."

The next part is staying motivated. For years, I had it in my head that exercising meant going to the gym, and not having fun. Then I realized that the main reason I wasn't exercising was that going to the gym was miserable.

I then began to look for ways to get moving that actually provided me with some enjoyment. My wife and I both love to hike, so we started hiking on the weekends. We recently moved to the Pacific Northwest and discovered that there are biking trails here as well. Riding a bike through the beautiful mountain scenery of the Cascades and the surrounding foothills is more than enjoyable for me.

Since I've started biking, I've been able to stay motivated to keep exercising. That's the secret to staying motivated. Find some sort of exercise that you actually enjoy doing, and do that. Even if it's just walking around the neighborhood. Experiment with what works for you, and soon you'll be able to establish your own exercise routine.

Another bit of useful information to help you stay motivated to work out is that it doesn't matter if you do one 60-minute workout per day or break it up into smaller 5 or 10 minute increments multiple times per day.

The Journal of the American Heart Association provided evidence in a 2018 study that mortality risk reductions associated with moderate to vigorous physical activity are independent of how activity is accumulated. In other words, if you do one longer workout per day or several shorter workouts per day, the results are the same.

So get up from your desk once every hour or so and do five or ten minutes of brisk walking. Over the course of the day it adds up.

Weighing Yourself

I'm going to tell you something different from what most diet programs tell you. You should weigh yourself every day. But...you should only weigh yourself every day if you can give yourself permission not to beat yourself up or feel guilty about what the scales say.

Your weight can fluctuate as much as five pounds per day, depending on your diet and fluid intake (see the *Water Intake* section below), so be aware of that should you choose to weigh yourself every day.

My reason for weighing every day is simple. The more data points you have, the more information you have. The more information you have, the easier it is to make changes.

If you weigh yourself every day, you have more data to use in modifying your relationship with food. Should you choose to weigh yourself every day,

I recommend doing it first thing in the morning, before drinking any coffee or eating breakfast. That's the best way to get a baseline weight, because first thing in the morning you've been fasting all night and your weight won't be influenced by any food or liquids.

Once you've weighed yourself, you may wish to record it in your Food Tracker or just make a mental note of it. If you find yourself feeling guilty or depressed because of what you see on the scales on a daily basis, then you're probably not ready to record your weight daily yet.

If that's the case, step back and only weigh yourself once per week or once per month. Continue to practice your mindful skills until you are able to weigh yourself daily without placing any judgments on the results.

Water Intake

In 2005 Sawka et al determined that a daily water intake of 3.7 liters for adult men and 2.7 liters for adult women meets the needs of the vast majority of persons. However, strenuous physical exercise and heat stress can greatly increase daily water needs. Drinking water regularly can also ease hunger pangs and make you feel more full with less food.

I make it a daily practice to fill my water bottle in the morning and keep it by my desk all day. Whenever I feel a craving to nibble on something at my desk, I take a sip of water instead. Not only does this help me control my appetite, but it keeps me hydrated throughout the day.

One word of caution about water...just be aware of how it influences your weight. It's better to weigh yourself first thing in the morning before drinking any water, coffee, or other liquids. The reason for this is that two 8-ounce cups of coffee will add one pound to your weight. Most people drink cups of coffee far bigger than 8 ounces.

The average 20-ounce coffee from most coffee shops will add almost a pound and a half to your weight! So if you weigh yourself after your morning coffee, you're getting skewed results.

Also be aware of your water intake throughout the day and how it might influence your weight. If you drink the recommended 64 ounces of water per day, that will add around 4 pounds to your weight for the day, and that doesn't even factor in any food you might eat during the day and how it might influence your weight.

If you stay hydrated and drink a healthy amount of water every day, just be aware that your weight may fluctuate as much as five or six pounds throughout the day. Don't panic if this happens. It's just water weight.

Six Common Traps and How to Avoid Them

There are six common reasons people "relapse" and return to their former eating habits after completing the Natural Eating program. The good news is that should one of these things appear in your life, you can turn it around using your mindful skills, and return to Natural Eating. Let's talk about what these things are and how to deal with them.

   1.   *Feelings of Guilt or Self-Blame*

The main problem with feelings of guilt or self-blame is that such feelings don't solve anything, and they can quite often make things worse. Guilt is the trigger to the binge-eating cycle.

Whenever you feel tempted to feel guilty or to blame yourself for something, instead of reaching for a comfort food, use your mindful skills to "ride the wave" until the feeling subsides.

   2.   *Unrealistic Expectations for Yourself or Others*

When people give up an addiction they justly expect for their life to improve. Giving up alcohol and drugs is a vital step, but it is just the beginning, there is much work to be done. And it's common for us to expect instant gratification. That's what we as addicts do!

So, when things aren't going our way (read: not improving fast enough for us) we think they'll never get better so, might as well go out and get high.

As for expectations of others, we addicts often have low expectations for ourselves but high expectations for everyone else. This way of thinking is destructive because it always leads to disappointment and pain. Nobody is perfect, and it is not right for adults to rely too much on other people.

3.   *Blaming Others*

This manifests as expecting others to take responsibility for your eating habits.

For example, suppose you're out to dinner with your spouse and he orders a huge dessert, then eats the entire thing in front of you. It'd be easy to do the same, and then say, "I couldn't help myself...it was his fault for tempting me."

The way around this is another mindful skill...having the wisdom to know what you can change and what you have to accept. You can't change other people, you can only change yourself. The danger here is when we fall into the trap of expecting others to take responsibility for changing us. That's an easy way to avoid taking responsibility for changing ourselves.

If you feel tempted to engage in blaming others, you can use your mindful skill of being non-judgmental and setting aside the blaming, shaming and guilt-tripping, and looking for solutions instead using your mindful skill of being effective (intentional).

4. *Emotional Eating*

One of the more difficult changes to make is the shift from emotional eating to dealing with problem emotions in other ways. In my own personal experience, the tendency to reach for comfort foods is like a wolf at your door.

As long as you remember the wolf is there, you're okay. But the moment you forget about the wolf is the moment he pounces. Likewise, the temptation to reach for comfort foods is always there because emotional eating is often easier than dealing with problem emotions in other ways.

It's easier to swallow our feelings than it is to swallow our pride and admit we need some help coping with our feelings, but if we can remember to use our mindful skills to shift from doing to being, and we can learn to just be with the feeling without trying to make it go away, then eventually we can master this skill and conquer the tendency to engage in emotional eating.

5. *Abusing Other Substances*

This comes up quite a bit, especially when someone decides to quit smoking and change their eating habits at the same time. Nicotine is an appetite depressant, and quitting smoking generally means an increase in appetite. This can also spill over into other substances, such as diet pills, or even amphetamines, in an attempt to control appetite through substance use or abuse.

The mindful way to deal with this issue is to recognize that there is a difference between appetite and hunger, and people generally engage in substance abuse as a way of dealing with appetite, not hunger. If this is an issue for you, you may wish to review the hunger vs.

appetite skills in *Lesson 6 Conscious Eating*.

6. *Apathy*

Once you gain more practice and skill with Natural Eating, it's natural to become confident in your ability to maintain healthy eating habits. The danger arises when you become overconfident or apathetic. This might manifest as mindless eating instead of conscious eating.

If this happens to you, remember that it's okay to be human. We all stumble from time to time. Just don't use that as an excuse to become apathetic or tell yourself "I can't do this." You are always free to start again.

FOOD TRACKER

You might consider adding a "weight" column to your Food Tracker so you can record your weight on a daily basis. You may then use this data to observe the relationship between what you eat and how it changes your weight.

Pay particular attention to the amount of fat and calories in each food item for the day, and how it might impact your weight the next day. Keep tracking this information over time and you will have a good road map towards eating the foods you love while maintaining a healthy weight.

KEY POINTS TO REMEMBER FROM LESSON 12

- If you believe you can do it, you will succeed.

- Don't rely on it as your sole means of controlling your weight.

- Exercise because it's good for you, and not because you want to lose weight.

- If you weigh yourself every day, do it first thing in the morning, before drinking any coffee or eating breakfast.

- If you drink the recommended 64 ounces of water per day, that will add 4 pounds to your weight for the day.

- Your weight may fluctuate as much as five pounds or more throughout the day.

- There are six common reasons people "relapse" and return to their former eating habits after completing the Natural Eating program. The good news is that should one of these things appear in your life, you can turn it around using your mindful skills, and return to Natural Eating.

REFERENCES

Cox, Carla. (2017). Role of Physical Activity for Weight Loss and Weight Maintenance. *Diabetes Spectrum*. 30. 157-160. 10.2337/ds17-0013.

Journal of the American Heart Association
Moderate-to-Vigorous Physical Activity and All-Cause Mortality: Do Bouts Matter?
https://www.ahajournals.org/doi/10.1161/JAHA.117.007678

Sawka, Michael & Cheuvront, Samuel & Carter, Robert. (2005). Human Water Needs. *Nutrition reviews*. 63. S30-9.

ABOUT THE AUTHOR

Charlton (Chuck) Hall is the current Executive Director of the Mindful Ecotherapy Center, LLC (www.mindfulecotherapy.org). He is a retired Marriage and Family Therapy Supervisor, a former (now retired) Registered Play Therapy Supervisor, and a Certified Hypnotherapist.

Chuck's area of research and interest is using Mindfulness and Ecotherapy to facilitate acceptance and change strategies within a family systemic 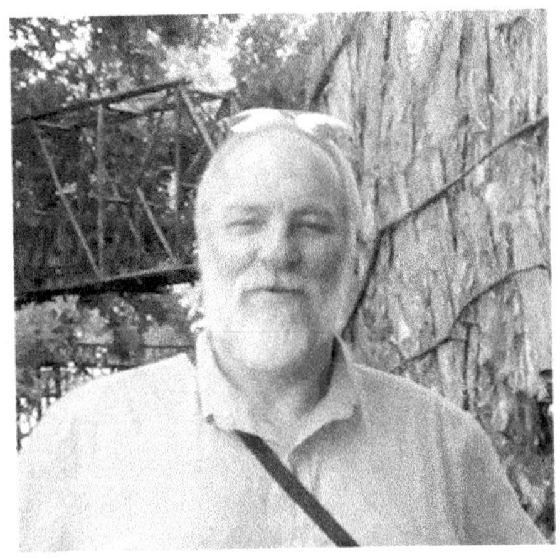 framework, and he has presented research at several conferences and seminars on this and other topics. Chuck's approach to therapy involves helping individuals and families to facilitate change through mindfulness and ecotherapy techniques in a non-judgmental, patient-centered, positive environment.

BOOKS BY CHARLTON HALL, PhD

The Mindfulness-Based Ecotherapy Workbook

This new version of the handbook introduces the 12 skills of Mindfulness-Based Ecotherapy (MBE) and introduces one of these skills at each of the 12 sessions in the program. Although this book is designed to accompany the 12-week Mindfulness-Based Ecotherapy workshop series, it may also be completed on your own at home. The experiential nature of the work allows anyone with access to outdoor spaces the opportunity to complete the series. If you are interested in participating in a workshop series near you, you can visit the Mindful Ecotherapy Center's website at www.mindfulecotherapy.org. The website contains a directory of Mindfulness-Based Ecotherapy programs worldwide at https://mindfulecotherapy.org/directory-2

Ecoplay: Re-Introducing Your Children to Nature

Ecoplay is an evidence-based eight-session training program designed to give parents and their children the opportunity for experiential activities outdoors that combine mindfulness, ecopsychology and the skills of positive parenting. Ecoplay is an authoritative, rather than authoritarian, approach to discipline and parenting. It is a framework for guiding your child(ren) to reconnect to nature in healing ways. Ecoplay trains parents to be nature-based play therapy facilitators for their own children. It is also a theoretical framework and approach to parenting that allows children to express themselves in play, their natural language. Ecoplay allows this expressive play to happen in healthy natural outdoor environments.

www.ingramcontent.com/pod-product-compliance
Lightning Source LLC
Chambersburg PA
CBHW060100260726
48658CB00004B/1351